Management of Acute and Chronic Diarrhea in Children

Fourth Edition

Management of Acute and Chronic Diarrhea in Children

Fourth Edition

Dr. S.K. Mittal
Head, Deptt. of Pediatrics & Chief Pediatric Gastroenterologist,
Max Hospital, Pitampura

Formerly, Director, Prof. & Head, Deptt. of Pediatrics,
Maulana Azad Medical College, New Delhi

CBS

CBS PUBLISHERS & DISTRIBUTORS
NEW DELHI • BANGALORE

ISBN : 81-239-1277-3

First Edition : 1992
Reprint : 1993
Second Edition : 1999
Reprint : 2000
Third Edition : 2003
Reprint : 2005
Fourth Edition : 2007

Published by :
S.K. Jain for CBS Publishers & Distributors,
4596/1A, 11, Darya Ganj, New Delhi-110 002 (India)
E-mail : cbspubs@vsnl.com
Website : www.cbspd.com

Publishing Director : Vinod K. Jain

Branch Office :
Seema House, 2975, 17th Cross, K.R. Road,
Bansankari 2nd Stage, Bangalore - 560070
Fax : 080-26771680 E-mail : cbsbng@vsnl.net

Printed at :
Chaman Enterprises, New Delhi - 110 002

Preface to the Fourth Edition

Last few years have seen revolutionary changes in management of diarrhea in children. Ultimate replacement of conventional WHO ORS by an hypo-osmolar ORS after years of worldwide research; recent discovery of role of zinc in acute and persistent diarrhea and continuing search for and additions of newer anti-secretory drugs and probiotics in the Indian pharmocopia has helped to propagate these changes.

Even in the field of chronic diarrhea, wider availability of serological tests and duodenal biopsy for diagnosis of celiac disease has helped to diagnose this condition early in larger number of children. Thus it was felt necessary to revise this book to incorporate latest changes. The whole of text has been carefully reviewed and the available new knowledge has been incorporated within the existing format. Emphasis has largely been in giving practical guidelines, incorporating the latest advances. A few references have also been added.

Dr. S.K. Mittal
Head, Deptt. of Pediatrics &
Chief Pediatric Gastroenterologist
Max Hospital, Pitampura
Formerly, Director, Prof. & Head,
Deptt. of Pediatrics,
Maulana Azad Medical College,
New Delhi

Preface to the First Edition

Diarrheal diseases still constitute a major component of practitioner's day to day work. In the absence of practical guidelines, an average practitioner finds himself greatly constrained in planning a rational management as he is unable to get many investigations which most text continue to advocate. He is thus forced to use treatment which may appear irrational by modern concepts of diarrheal disease management.

A few of my lecture notes on management of acute diarrhea, meant for the practitioners, were published by Delhi Branch of I.M.A. College of General Practitioners in August 1989 in a manuscript entitled "Drugs, Diet & Fluid in Diarrhea". In this hand book not only these three articles have been updated but a few chapters have also been added on the problems of persistent diarrhea which is assuming greater importance in clinical practice. The style of these essays have remained the same and the effort is largely to outline a practical approach in the management of diarrheal diseases which has been found useful in our clinical practice.

The discussion of pathogenetic mechanisms have been interwoven into the practical approach so that the practitioners can understand the rationale of each approach.

The texts are briefly referenced with a view to stimulate at least some of the practitioners to read more about these problems and to understand them even better.

I hope the practitioners would find the book useful and would be able to apply the knowledge gained, in their day to day practice with ultimate goal of improving child health.

Dr. S.K. Mittal
Assoc. Professor
Department of Pediatrics
Maulana Azad Medical College
New Delhi

Contents

1

Acute Diarrhea

AN OVERVIEW

Most diarrheal episodes in children are self limiting in nature requiring only replacement of fluids for prevention and treatment of dehydration. Hence in all management protocols, emphasis has largely been on rehydration. Prior to the discovery of oral rehydration, reliance was largely placed on intravenous rehydration which obviously put a large strain on health resources and was quite often out of reach of many a children living in remote areas. Advent of oral rehydration therapy has greatly revolutionized the management of diarrheal dehydration, making it possible to provide a full and satisfactory treatment at home itself, in large majority of childhood diarrheal episodes. However, there remains a significant proportion of children who require not only appropriate drugs for their management but may also require intravenous rehydration. It is important to be able to decide on clinical grounds as to which child would require drugs and which child would require intravenous fluids. The clinician should also be able to choose a drug appropriately and also to administer intravenous fluids rationally.

Further, recent advances in our understanding of pathogenic mechanisms of diarrhea and of the nutrient absorptive functions of the gut during and after a diarrheal episode, has almost completely revolutionized traditional views of feeding in diarrheal disease management.

Many newer drugs like racecadotril, probiotics, various preparations of zinc etc. continue to be introduced with tall claims of efficacy in acute diarrhea.

An average practitioner is hard put to understand these changes in management protocols or to understand the exact role of newer drugs, and to incorporate them in his clinical practice. The following approach has been developed as a mean to help him arrive at a rational management protocol, incorporating results of latest research.

What is Diarrhea?

For epidemiological purposes diarrhea is defined as passage of 3 or more loose stools per day. However, this definition may not be strictly applicable in infants where it is more prudent to consider diarrhea when the child has a sudden increase in frequency of less formed stools. Green/yellow colour of stool does not necessarily mean that the child is having diarrhea. Acute diarrhea is defined as diarrhea of less than 7 days duration.

"Diarrheal Episodes" which are not Diarrhea

Before the approach to a child with acute diarrhea is discussed it is important to remember certain clinical situations in which the child (more likely an infant) may be brought in for "diarrhea" but actually has no diarrhea. Some of these situations are given below :

(i) **Transitional stools of the newborn :** All newborns pass frequent and semiformed or watery greenish yellow stools between 2nd and 5th to 7th day of life. At this age most newborns also have some weight loss. This is often interpreted as diarrhea by the uninitiated. This represents transition from black (dark green) meconium to golden yellow stools of breast fed babies. It is self limiting and requires no treatment.

(ii) **Gastro colic pattern :** Young infants upto 3-6 months of age very often pass a stool immediately after a feed. Breast milk fed babies even normally have watery to semi-liquid stools. Breast-fed infant may pass as many as 8-10 stools per day almost after each feed. This is due to exaggerated gastro-colic pattern at this age. This pattern occurs quite normally and is even more apt to occur after an attack of acute infectious diarrhea. Often this is interpreted as unsuitability of breast milk or cow's milk. Breast feeding is unnecessarily stopped or cow's milk withdrawn or diluted, leading to malnutrition.

This requires no treatment as such. Supplementing with semi-solid foods after 3-4 months of age would help in improving the symptoms.

(iii) **Involuntary passage of stools in a constipated child.** Quite often a child (between 3-6 yrs. of age) is brought in with complaints of passing small watery stools involuntarily in the undergarments. This may happen 3-4 times a day and parents may think that the child is having diarrhea. However, these children have underlying constipation with "overflow incontinence", because of stretch of anal sphincter due to chronically retained stools. A rectal examination will confirm the diagnosis of retained stools with a loaded rectum. Treatment would be required for constipation and not for diarrhea.

Epidemiological Aspects of Diarrhea—Predisposing Factors

Diarrheal disease still constitute one of the most important cause of morbidity and mortality in childhood. Globally over 1 billion episodes of diarrhea occur every year. Among children, in India, an average under 5 child gets 2-3 episodes of diarrhea each year and it is estimated that over 200 million episodes of diarrhea occur each year. In urban slum areas, under five children may get upto 6-8 episodes per year. Despite widespread use of ORS, it is still believed that diarrheal disease accounts for almost 1 million under 5 deaths in our country every year.

Malnutrition is also very frequent. About 53% of under five children are malnourished in our country and 1.5% are severely malnourished. As malnutrition has an adverse impact on the frequency, severity and outcome of diarrheal diseases, malnutrition and diarrhea constitute a particularly bad mix and they together become the largest cause of mortality in under five children.

Etiological Factors in Acute Diarrhea

Acute diarrhea can occur because of gastrointestinal infection due to a variety of infecting organisms (Table 1.1). Large majority of diarrheas are due to Rota virus, pathogenic strains of E. coli, V. cholerae and Shigella.

Apart from infection, food intolerance to various foods/food

Table 1.1. Etiological aspects of diarrhea

G.I. infection	
Viral	Rota, Norwalk, Astro virus, Entero virus
Bacterial	ETEC, EPEC, V. cholera, Shigella, Salmonella, Yersina, Campylobacter
Parasite	Amebiasis, Giardia, H. nana, Candida
Fungal	Candida
Food intolerance	Lactose intolerance
	Cow's milk protein intolerance
	Gluten intolerance
Systemic infections	Otitis media, pneumonia, meningitis, urinary tract infection etc.

components like lactose, cow's milk protein, gluten (protein in wheat) can also cause diarrhea. This intolerance may be due to inability to metabolize and absorb the substance (like lactose) or due to a hypersensitivity to the particular protein, resulting in immune mediated damage to the small bowel mucosa and subsequent diarrhea. Intolerance due to different proteins would require complete withdrawal of offending protein from the diet.

Systemic infections can also cause diarrhea and vomiting mimicking an attack of acute gastro enteritis. This is most likely to occur among infants (< 1 yr. of age). This has been labelled as parenteral diarrhea or diarrhea with associated infection. Thus infections like otitis media, pneumonia, meningitis, urinary tract infection etc. can lead to diarrhea. Here the treatment is basically targeted to the systemic infection (e.g. Ampicilin/amoxycillin for otitis media).

Pathogenetic Mechanism of Acute Diarrhea

Different organisms cause acute diarrhea due to variety of pathogenetic mechanism.

Rota virus (and other viruses) : They cause jejunal mucosal damage resulting in villous atrophy and interruption in absorptive mechanisms. As lactase enzyme is maximally present in superficial layer of villi, a transient lactose intolerance may also be seen. The mucosal damage is maximum at the onset of illness and starts recovering within 24-36 hours. Resulting diarrhea is severe and watery type.

Vibrio cholerae : This gram –ve bacillus releases entero-toxin (which is heat labile). This enterotoxin acts on the chloride secretory mechanism in the small intestine by stimulating cyclic AMP (Adenosine Monophosphate), through activation of adenylate cyclase enzyme.

Vibrio toxin is a powerful toxin which causes severe secretery (watery) diarrhea with or without vomiting. It is self limiting in nature, if the lost fluids can be replaced adequately.

Esch coli : Only a few strains of Esch coli cause diarrhea. Some of the strains release enterotoxin and cause toxigenic diarrhea much in the same manner as Vibrio cholerae. The strains are called entertoxigenic Esch coli (ETEC). There are some other strains which have been epidemiologically related to diarrheal illness but they do not liberate any toxins. They are called Enteropathogenic Esch coli (EPEC). Exact mechanism of diarrhea due to EPEC is not known.

ETEC strains release heat labile (LT) and/or heat stable (ST) enterotoxin. Heat labile enterotoxin released by ETEC is structurally similar and acts similarly to the cholera toxin. ST causes diarrhea by stimulating guanyl cyclase with an associated increase in cyclic GMP. This again causes severe secretory diarrhea.

Diarrhea caused by EPEC/ETEC strains are not associated with any structural damage to intestinal mucosa. They also largely cause self limiting illness. Antibiotics have no role in their management.

Shigella : Various serotypes cause diarrhea by causing invasive illness of the large bowel. There is extensive damage and inflammation of colonic mucosa, resulting in exudative (mucus, blood) diarrhea. The organism actually invade the mucosa and cause acute inflammation.

Some strains of shigella may also liberate exotoxins (Shiga toxin) which causes severe systemic toxemia including high fever, convulsions which may occasionally precede the onset of diarrheal illness.

Rarely shigella infection may even manifest as watery diarrhea, at least initially due to liberation of enterotoxin which acts on the intestinal mucosa much in the same manner as enterotoxin of Esch. coli.

Severe shigellosis may also be associated with hemolytic-uremic syndrome manifesting as hemolytic anemia, thrombocytopenia and uremia.

Approach to a Child with Acute Diarrhea

When a child presents with acute diarrhea, the treating physician must remember that diarrhea is *only a symptom.* It is neither a disease *per se* nor a diagnosis in itself. Like any other symptom (e.g. fever) it can be caused by a variety of factors (Table 1.1) and it is for the clinician to make the underlying diagnosis which is responsible for the particular episode of diarrhea. The most important clue to the underlying cause is provided by a carefully taken history and a thorough physical examination. Simple investigations like routine stool examination and a differential leucocyte count may occasionally be required but other investigations are as a rule neither required nor useful.

History in a Case of Acute Diarrhea

The type and character of loose stool is of major importance. The frequency, colour, consistency, content (mucus or blood) etc. provide important clues. On the basis of consistency and content, one can classify the child to be having watery, mucoid or bloody (invasive) diarrhea.

Clinically it is useful to view acute diarrheal diseases as either *acute watery diarrhea* or as an *acute invasive (or bacillary dysentry) diarrhea* syndrome. Presence of frank blood in loose stools, makes it a case of invasive diarrhea. All other cases are grouped as watery diarrhea syndrome. Etiological agents associated with there two types of acute diarrhea syndrome are listed in Table 1.2.

Although age and associated symptoms can help in distinguishing the underlying cause of acute diarrhea of different types but

Table 1.2. Etiological Factors in Different Types of Acute Diarrheal Syndromes

Watery Diarrhea/Mucoid Diarrhea
• Rota virus and other viral diarrheas
• ETEC, *V. Cholerae, Campylobacter*, EPEC
• Parenteral Infections (Otitis media, U.T.I., Pneumonia)
• Giardia (Occasionally)
• Early stages of *Shigella* (rarely)
Invasive Diarrhea (Loose stools with blood)
• *Shigella,* Enteroinvasive *E. coli*, Enterohemorrhagic E. coli
• *Salmonella* (nontyphoidal)
• *Campylobacter*
• *Yersinia*

clinically it is usually not required as rational management can be planned on the basis of syndromatic (watery or invasive diarrhea) diagnosis without precise microbiological diagnosis.

Green stools

Common man associates passage of green stools with presence of (bacterial) gut infection. But that is not necessarily so. Passage of green stools, only means intestinal hurry which may or may not be due to GI infection. *Per se* they do not indicate the need of antibiotics.

Fever in Acute Diarrhea

Presence of fever in a child with acute diarrhea needs special evaluation. Fever in Rota virus infection can occasionally be high grade but the child almost never looks toxic. In shigellosis (stools mucoid or bloody), child has fever and toxemia and pus cells in stool. Parenteral infections cause not only fever but other symptoms like excessive crying (otitis media, meningitis), respiratory distress (pneumonitis) and dysuria or urinary frequency (U.T.I.). Children with fever and diarrhea thus deserve a thorough examination. However, presence or height of fever by itself, does not necessarily suggest a bacterial infection and should not be an indication to start antibiotics.

As gastrointestinal infections (except *Salmonella*) *per se*, rarely cause fever beyond 36-48 hours, every child with fever of more than 48 hours duration, need all the investigations as for a case of pyrexia. *As a rule, diarrhea is of secondary importance in a child with persistent fever*. Again onset of fever preceding the onset of diarrhea should also warrant search for a systemic infection.

Vomiting in Acute diarrhea

Vomiting occurs frequently in children with acute diarrhea but usually does not provide any etiological clue. Although it is more frequent in Rota virus infection and toxigenic (*V. Cholera*, ETEC) diarrheas, but it can occur in diarrheal disease of any etiology. It's only significance is that it may occasionally interfere with successful application of oral rehydration.

It should, however, be remembered that a child with isolated or persistent vomiting usually has an affliction outside the gastrointestinal tract (throat, chest, meninges, liver, urinary tract etc.) rather than in the gastrointestinal tract itself. Hence, all children with persistent vomitings (with or without diarrhea) need very careful appraisal for these problems, rather than just action to stop vomiting.

Physical Examination

In a child with acute diarrhea, thorough physical examination is required with special reference to:

(a) Hydration status.
(b) Nutritional status (weight, mid arm circumference).
(c) Presence of parenteral infection, if any.

Hydration Status

As dehydration is the single most important cause of morbidity and mortality in acute diarrhea, assessment of severity of dehydration is of utmost importance (Table 1.3). Choice of fluid therapy is determined by the severity of dehydration.

Table 1.3. Assessment of Dehydration

	Degree of wt. loss	*Features*
Mild	3-5%	Increased thirst, irritability
Moderate	6-10%	Skin turgor, depressed fontanelle, dry mucous membranes, sunken eyes, decreased urine output
Severe	> 10%	Drowsy, apathetic, refusal to feed/drink, anuria, acidosis, shock

Most infants and children with mild to moderate dehydration can be safely managed with oral rehydration therapy alone, therefore, from management point of view, mild and moderate dehydration can be clubbed together and termed as "*some*" dehydration (as per WHO classification).

Clinically it is important to distinguish children with severe dehydration from those with *some* (mild/moderate) dehydration. Assessment of sensorium is very helpful for this. While children with some dehydration are irritable but they are alert and keen to drink fluids. On the other hand, severely dehydrated children are drowsy, apathetic and unwilling to drink fluids. Change of sensorium in severe dehydration sets in even before, the signs and symptoms of shock and should be carefully looked for.

If premorbid weight is available, then the degree of weight loss is the most sensitive indicator of diarrheal dehydration. Of course if symptoms/signs of shock are present then irrespective of presence or absence of any other feature, the child should be managed as a case of severe dehydration.

Nutritional Status

Nutritional status is now recognised as one of the important determinant of diarrheal duration and diarrheal mortality even much more so since the discovery and widespread application of oral rehydration therapy. ORT has decreased deaths due to dehydration thus bringing into focus nutritional status as a contributor of mortality. Body weight is the most important indicator of nutritional status and plotting it on a "Road to Health" chart will immediately tell the severity of malnutrition. In malnourished children with diarrhea, apart from a serious search for focus of infection outside the gastrointestinal tract, action is also warranted for early nutritional supplementation. While children with body weight between 60-80% of the expected (mild to moderate malnutrition) can usually be managed like normal nourished children, with extra attention to nutritional intake; children with diarrhea and severe malnutrition (< 60% body weight) would usually require hospitalisation.

Parenteral Infection and Diarrhea

As parenteral infections often cause diarrhea in children esp. in infants, it is important to carefully screen children with diarrhea for parenteral infections. In this regard, availability and use of an otoscope is of utmost importance to diagnose cases of otitis media which frequently present with acute diarrhea.

The following features should alert a clinician to the possibility of a parenteral infection in an infant with diarrhea:

a) Fever preceding the onset of diarrhea, or persisting for more than 48 hours. Degree of fever is not important.

b) Severe malnutrition (body wt. < 60%). The symptoms and signs of systemic infection may often be absent in malnourished children.
c) Lethargy, inactivity *in absence of dehydration* or persisting even after correction of dehydration.
d) Signs/symptoms of parenteral infection e.g. bulging fontanelle, excessive cry, respiratory distress, ear ache, burning micturition etc.
e) Dehydration persisting or recurring despite adequate fluid replacement.

As infants are much more likely to have associated parenteral infection with diarrheal episodes, even more careful search should be made for infection among infants with diarrhea. Frequency of systemic infection in malnourished children with diarrhea is so high that it is now recommended that all these children should get systemic antibiotics.

Investigations

In normal nourished children with watery diarrhea, no fever and no dehydration, no investigations are required. They can be managed as per Fig. 1.1.

Stool Microscopy

Children with watery diarrhea having fever and/or dehydration and children with mucoid diarrhea, deserve a microscopic examination of freshly passed stool (Table 1.4). If more than 10 pus cells per high power field are present, then a possibility of invasive diarrhea is strong and these children need management on the lines (see Fig. 1.2) of bacillary dysentry.

Children with frank bloody diarrhea do not require stool examination as the diagnosis (of invasive diarrhea) is clear. However, if blood does not disappear even after 48 hours of suitable antibiotic

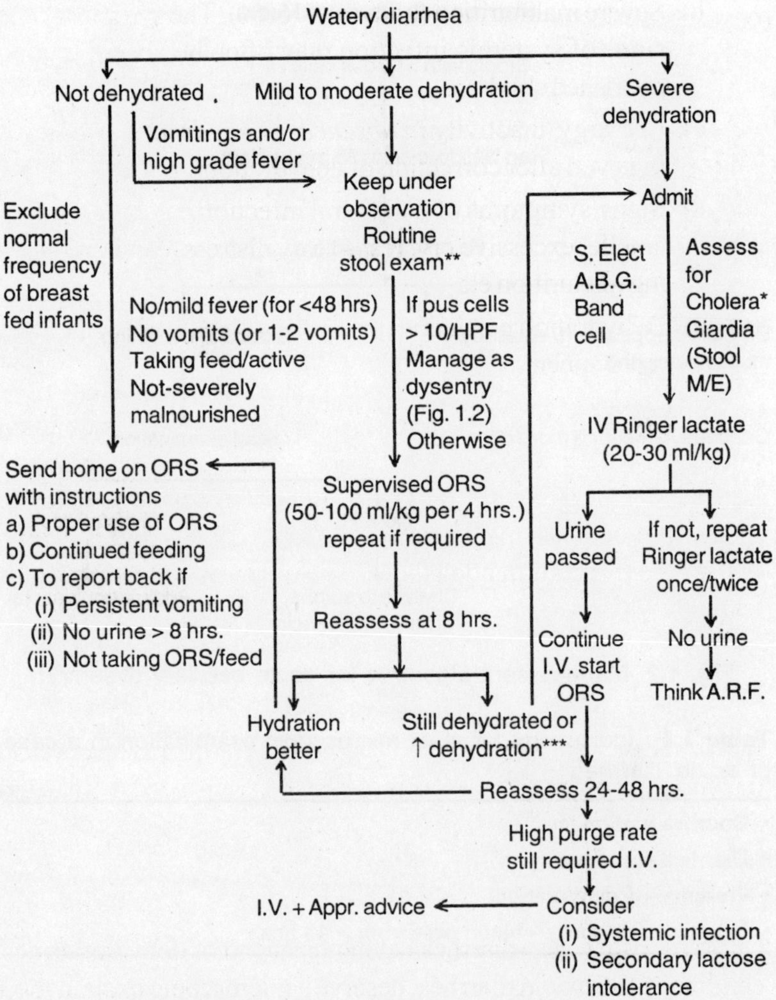

N.B. *(a) Suspect and manage as cholera if rapid onset of dehydration in a short time, irrespective of stool character (see text)

**(b) Routine stool microscopy in all admitted children for (i) Pus cells, (ii) V. Cholera, (iii) Giardia trophozoites

***(c) Carefully look for systemic infection specially in : (i) Infants, (ii) Severely malnourished, (iii) Persistent (>48 hrs.) pyrexia, (iv) Toxic/lethargic child. Consider appropriate antimicrobials (see text)

(d) Obtain serum electrolytes and ABG (if available) for those requiring I.V. See also Fig. 2.2, p. 57.

Fig. 1.1. Management algorithm for acute watery diarrhea.

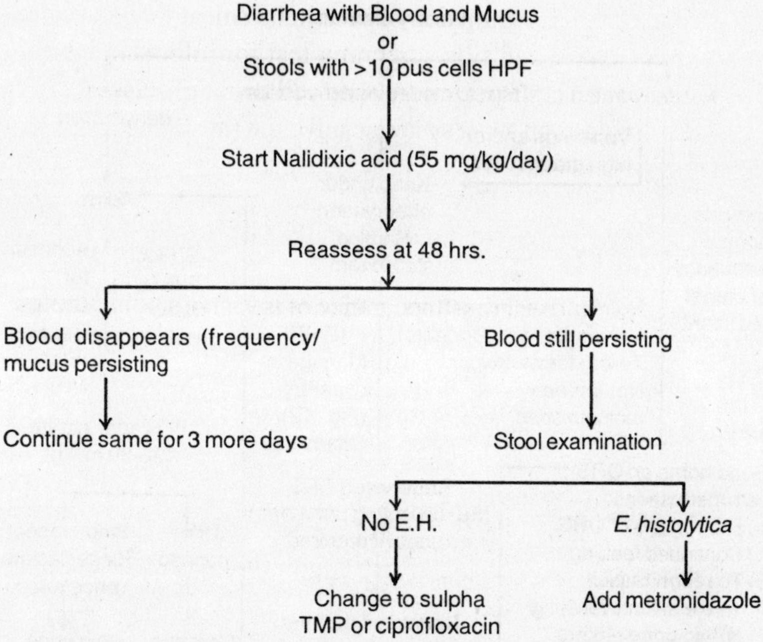

Fig. 1.2. Management algorithm for acute bacillary dysentry.

Table 1.4 : Indications for stool microscopic examination in a case of acute diarrhea

- Diarrhea with mucus
- Diarrhea with fever
- Presence of dehydration
- In cases of dysentry - blood persisting > 48 hrs.

therapy, then it may be worth doing a routine microscopic examination of stool to rule out an occasional case of acute amebiasis.

Investigations for Systemic Infections

Appropriate investigations (urine routine, culture, blood culture, X-ray chest, C.S.F. etc.) may be required whenever systemic infection is suspected (localising signs/symptoms, malnutrition and/or persistent pyrexia). Examination of peripheral smear for band cells has proved a useful bed side screening test for infants in whom systemic infection is suspected. A band cell count of > 20% of the neutrophils suggests an acute systemic infection (in absence of acute dysentry).

Sigmoidoscopy

In hospitalized children, first appearance of invasive stools denotes either a hospital-acquired gut infection (usually *Salmonella typhimurium*) or a much more severe condition called antibiotic colitis or pseudomembranous colitis (occuring in those on broad-spectrum antibiotics). An early sigmoidoscopy may therefore be a worthwhile investigation in these cases to distinguish between the two. Also sigmoidoscopy will be indicated if bloody diarrhea (colitis) is persistent, to rule out other rare conditions like amoebic colitis, ulcerative colitis etc.

Stool Cultures

Stool cultures are practically of no value in the clinical management of children with diarrhea. Children with frank blood in stool require management on the lines of shigellosis and hence stool cultures are not required. In other cases isolation of a bacterial organism or its antibiotics sensitivity has no significance whatsoever in management.

The diagnosis of cholera should be made clinically and can be confirmed by microscopic examination for motile bacteria. Culture may be required for epidemiological purposes rather than clinical usefulness. Mere isolation of a bacterial organism like *Esch. coli, Klebsiella* etc. does not indicate that it is the responsible pathogen as they are often cultured from normal stools also. In any case, there is no role of any antibiotic or chemotherapeutic agents for these bacterial organism isolated from diarrheal stools. Thus stool organisms (except in shigellosis) or their sensitivity should never be determinant of the choice of antibiotic in a case of diarrhea.

Thus it is obvious that most children with acute diarrhea can rationally and scientifically be managed on the basis of clinical assessment alone. The algorithm presented (Fig. 1.1 & 1.2) will serve as a helpful guide in decision making at various stages of clinical management of children with acute diarrhea.

MANAGEMENT

Fig. 1.1 and 1.2 outline the approach to the management of children with watery/mucoid and invasive diarrheas respectively. It will be noted that in most cases, rational management decisions can be taken and carried out successfully on the basis of clinical assessment alone. As pointed above, only in a few cases, who have fever, significant dehydration and/or mucoid diarrhea, a stool microscopic examination is warranted.

SUMMARY

After thorough clinical appraisal a child with diarrhea can be classified in one of the following groups :

Watery diarrhea with no dehydration : More than 90% of children with watery diarrhea have no dehydration at initial presentation to a health facility/personnel. They can just be managed with additional home available fluids and O.R.S.

Watery diarrhea with some dehydration : About 8-9% of children with watery diarrhea have some dehydration. These children can be managed with oral rehydration *under supervision*.

Watery diarrhea with severe dehydration : About 1% of children with diarrhea develop severe dehydration. This would require intravenous fluids for rapid correction of shock/anuria and then hydration with ORS.

Acute dysentry/acute invasive diarrhea : These children would require appropriate antibiotics. Associated dehydration is management with oral dehydration. Early restoration of normal diet is even more important in these children.

Diarrhea with associated infection : Here the primary problem is systemic infection. Management is determined by the site and severity of systemic infection. The type of diarrhea may be watery or mucoid and very rarely invasive. Appropriate antibiotic for systemic infection is the mainstay of management with appropriate fluids intravenously or orally.

Young infants (< 1 year of age) and severe malnourished children are at great risk of developing diarrhea with associated systemic infection. Clinical manifestation (of systemic infection) may also not be very specific and these children require careful appraisal by a trained child specialist. These children are preferably managed in a hospital setting.

Details of management (drugs, diet and fluids) are discussed subsequently.

2

Drugs, Diet and Fluids in Diarrhea

Most texts on diarrhea management mention that "drugs are not useful in diarrhea and may even prolong the course of diarrheal illness". Alternatively they give a choice of drugs according to causative agents, like *Shigella*, *V. cholerae* etc., a factor, which is but rarely known in day to day practice. In absence of any definite guidelines based on clinical features and easily obtainable investigations, a practitioner is usually at a loss for the rational selection of drugs in a child with diarrhea. His confusion is even more marked as he sees that majority of consultant practitioners and even medical college teachers, continue to use age old irrational drug treatment in diarrheal children. Following are some practical guidelines to use the available drugs in a rational manner.

It needs to be re-emphasised that diarrhea (like fever) is only a symptom and not a disease per se. It can be caused by a number of factors and by different pathogenetic mechanisms. It is important to be able to delineate the underlying cause and to treat the same, rather than to take action for stopping the (symptom of) diarrhea. In any case, in large majority of cases, acute diarrhea is a self-limiting illness warranting nothing more than replacement of fluids. *It should be considered only as an attempt by the body to "flush out" the enteropathogens from the G.I. tract. As lots of fluids are lost in this flushing out process, the same should be replaced and no attempt need to be made to stop the "flushing out" process.*

As already pointed out, clinically a child with diarrhea, presents in three distinct manners :

(i) As watery diarrhea (liquid or semi-liquid stools, without mucus or blood).
(ii) As mucoid diarrhea (semiliquid or semiformed stools with mucus but no blood).
(iii) As invasive diarrhea or dysentery (loose stools with blood and/or mucus).

Watery Diarrhea

This is the most frequent clinical presentation and constitutes about 80% of all diarrheal episodes in children. Vomiting is often associated and occasionally fever is also present. Most cases of watery diarrhea are due to either viral infections or due to noninvasive bacterial (ETEC, EPEC etc.) infection. They do not require any drugs. However it is important to exclude cholera or associated systemic infection in these cases. With the help of clinical features mentioned in Table 2.1, it should be possible to make a probable diagnosis clinically in majority of cases and thus to plan rational drug therapy.

Clinical Identification of a Case of Cholera

Cholera cases can be identified clinically when a child older than 5 years of age presents with watery diarrhea (and vomiting) and severe dehydration of sudden onset. Typical case history is of a child who went to sleep after eating a dinner, and started having diarrhea and vomiting in the night and is brought to the hospital early in the

Table 2.1. Drugs in Watery Diarrhea

Condition	*Suspect*	*Confirm*	*Drugs*
Cholera	>5 yr*, sudden severe dehydration	Hanging drop** stool c/s	Doxycycline 6 mg/kg** once + ORS
Diarrhea with associated systemic infection	Infants/Severely malnourished children, features of systemic infection	TLC, DLC Band Cell urine R/E X-ray chest	Appropriate antibiotics + ORS
All other cases	Features of cholera and systemic infection absent	No need	Only ORS

* > 2 yrs. in endemic area, ** Not reliable unless performed very carefully, *** To prevent secondary cases. In younger children, chloramphenicol (50 mg/kg/day × 3 day) can be used.

morning with features of severe dehydration/shock. The stools are not characteristic and typical "rice water" stools are but uncommonly seen (< 30%), at least in childhood cholera. Single dose of doxycycline in children above 6 years of age is all that is required for clinically suspected cases of cholera. In younger children, chloramphenicol (50 mg/kg/d × 3 days) may be given.

Identification of Systemic Infection (Table 2.2)

Special attempts should be made to exclude parenteral infections by a thorough physical examination (ear drums, fontanelle, chest etc.). Characteristically infants with systemic infection and diarrhea have fever, look toxic and pass frequent, watery (with or without mucus) stools of low volume. In case of doubt, a blood examination for total and differential leucocyte count (esp. band cells) may be obtained to exclude the presence of systemic infection.

Rarely organisms like *Shigella* and non-typhoidal *salmonella* may also produce watery diarrhea in initial phases. Fever, toxemia etc. are usually marked and stool examination would usually dem-

Table 2.2. Associated Systemic Infection in Diarrhea

High Risk cases
- Infants (< 1 year)
- Severely malnourished children

Suspect if any one or more clinical feature present
- Fever prior to onset of diarrhea
- Fever persisting more than 48 hours
- Abnormal physical signs/symptoms
  excessive cry, respiratory distress, bulging fontanelle, congested ear drums
- Lethargy/Inactive esp. without significant dehydration
- Persistent or recurrent dehydration
- Diarrhea persisting beyond 7 days

onstrate the presence of pus cells in these cases. Also the band cell count is usually high (more than 15%). Diarrhea becomes frankly invasive within 24 to 36 hours. So, if a child with watery diarrhea has fever and a normal physical examination, it may be prudent to get a stool examination done for pus cells.

Drugs in Watery Diarrhea

Oral Rehydration Solution (ORS) : Major problem in children with watery diarrhea is loss of fluids and electrolytes and consequent dehydration. This loss, whether due to mucosal damage (Rota virus) or due to stimulation of secretory mechanisms (*ETEC, V. cholera*), is entirely self limiting and settles down within 3-5 days. Thus the only rational treatment for watery diarrhea is replacement of fluid and electrolytes, and for this oral rehydration solution is the best and probably the only drug, required in large majority of watery diarrhea cases. Its efficacy in preventing and curing dehydration has been proven beyond doubt (for details of oral rehydration see the section on Fluids & Electrolytes), *but it should be remembered that it is not a treatment of diarrhea but only of dehydration.*

Antibiotic & Chemotherapeutic agents : Majority of children with acute diarrhea neither have cholera nor associated systemic infection and do not require any drugs. Thus almost all infants and young children with watery diarrhea can be safely and scientifically managed with only oral fluid replacement. Fever and corryza are also often present in Rota virus infections and even in ETEC diarrhea and hence by themselves do not constitute indications for the use of antibiotics.

Although, it may appear axiomatic that no antibiotics need be given to children with bacterial (ETEC, EPEC) diarrhea, but this can be understood when one realises that the diarrhea in these children is due to action of toxins released by the bacteria rather than by the bacteria themselves (see pathogenetic mechanisms of acute diarrhea). Further, these bacteria remain only on superficial layers of mucosa and are not invasive in character and do not cause any structural damage to the intestine. Even in cases of cholera, the antibiotics are given to prevent the occurrence of secondary cases as the course of disease is totally unaffected by antibiotics in the patient himself.

However, presence of pus cells (> 10/HPF) in stools even in a case of watery diarrhea would warrant the use of appropriate chemotherapeutic agents on the lines of bacillary dysentery. Also, it is highly unusual for fever in a viral diarrhea to persist beyond 36-48 hours. So, a reappraisal of the child to carefully search for a focus of infection (outside the G.I. tract) is called for in such a situation. Urinary tract infection should be specially looked for in children with diarrhea and persistent fever. Presence of bandemia in peripheral smear (bands > 20% of total neutrophils) also suggests systemic infection.

Antisecretory agents : In an attempt to reverse process of active secretion induced by toxigenic bacteria (*ETEC, V. cholerae*) many drugs have been developed. Chlorpromazine, Salicylates, Loperamide, Indomethacin, Berberine, Clonidine, Somatostatin etc.

are some of these drugs, which in experimental animals have been shown to have some antisecretory effect. But clinical trials with their use have been largely disappointing. Reduction in secretions is not more than 15-20% and most of these drugs (chlorpromazine, loperamide) cause frequent and unacceptable side effects in doses required to achieve this reduction. Thus, while search for an effective anti-secretory agent continues, it is clear that as of today, none is available which can be considered safe and effective for clinical use.

Recently another potentially useful antisecretory drug has been introduced in the Indian markets for treatment of diarrhea. *Racecadotril* is a morphine analogue which acts by inhibiting enkephalinase enzyme, thus allowing enkephalins present in myentric plexus to exert their antisecretory affects. Its action is largely on the secretory mechanism of the gut and it has hardly any CNS action or action on the gut motility, thus it does not cause CNS side effects like sedation etc and also does not decrease gut motility, two dreaded side effects of other opioid analogs. It decreases intestinal secretions and has been shown to be effective in some studies in decreasing stool output in children with watery diarrhea, especially rota virus diarrhea.

Although the drug is licensed for use in India, no study is available from our country or other developing countries (except one from Peru) to support the routine use of this drug in acute watery diarrhea. It has not been effective in diarrhea due to *V. cholera*, which produces the most typical and most severe secretory diarrhea. Hypokalaemia can occur as a side effect with the use of the drug. Also its safety profile with prolonged or recurrent use especially in malnourished children is not well established.

Currently available evidence does not warrant its routine use in acute diarrhea. Till more studies are available demonstrating its safety and efficacy, it will not be wise to use this drug.

Antiemetics : Vomiting is a frequent and annoying, nay distressing problem, associated with diarrheal disease. Usually this is self limiting and a rational use of ORS (see under Fluid therapy) can help to control these in large majority of cases. Nevertheless an antiemetic may be warranted in some cases of acute gastroenteritis. It is safer to use drugs like metoclopropamide (0.5 mg/kg) or domperidone (0.3 mg/kg), rather than triflupromazine (siquil) or chlorpromazine (largactil) etc., which are much more toxic.

Drugs like odensterone are strong antiemetic drugs which act centrally by blocking five hydroxy tryptamine (serotonin) receptors without significant extrapyramidal side effects. They are basically recommended for prevention and control of vomiting due to anesthetic agents in post-operative stage or that due to cancer chemotherapy. Its use in general vomiting (as seen in gastritis, gastroentertitis) is not really justified. However, it may be used with caution. It may cause headache, dizziness and allergic reactions. It is not recommended if there is underlying liver dysfunction. It is also not recommended in children < 4 year of age.

Also if vomitings are not controlled even after one or two doses of the antiemetic, it would be important to do a repeat and thorough examination to look for an underlying extra gastrointestinal cause and consider intravenous fluid therapy. *Antiemetics should never be prescribed on a round-the-clock basis.*

Binding agents : Kaolin, pectin etc. have a doubtful therapeutic role and in controlled clinical trials have largely failed to give consistent benefits. These binding agents, including the antibiotic combinations with binding agents, have largely been banned in India.

Antimotility or antispasmodic drugs : Diphenoxylate, atropine, meperidon have been used in an attempt to decrease the annoying frequency or to provide relief to pain especially in colitis. But they have no effect on the basic pathogenetic mechanism i.e. excess of fluid and electrolyte losses, which continue despite apparent decrease in frequency. They may thus produce a false sense of well being. In fact, as increased intestinal motility is an essential host defense mechanism (for flushing out the toxins) to overcome diarrheal illness, the use of antimotility agents cannot be justified at all. They can also cause abdominal distension and paralytic ileus, which may even warrant hospitalization. These drugs potentiate *Shigella* infection and produce toxic colon. In general these drugs should not be used in children with diarrhea and their use is particularly contra-indicated if invasive diarrhea is suspected. Liquid preparations of these drugs have also been banned in India.

Probiotics in Diarrhea

Probiotics are a group of nutrition supplements which contain viable strains of certain microorganisms which promote the growth of normal microflora of the gut. As normal resident microflora of the gut has an important role to play in digestion and absorption of many nutrients and to keep the growth of pathogenic organisms at bay, these probiotics can be helpful in a variety of diarrhoeal disorders and other GI problems. These probiotics are usually found in abundance in foods which have undergone fermentation. Curd or yoghurt is a good source of probiotics as it is a rich source of Lactobacillus.

Sacchromyces boulardii, a fungus, and a variety of stains of bacteria like *Lactobacillus*, *Biofidobacter* and *Streptococcus* act as probiotics. In fact, more than a thousand strains of *Lactobacillus* exist and it is only a few of them which act as probiotics. For a strain to act as probiotic, it is essential that :

i) It should contain a large number of viable organisms till the time it is ingested.

ii) These viable organisms should be able to withstand the hostile acid environment of stomach and alkaline bile in the duodenum.

iii) After surving the above, it should be able to multiply in the jejunal/ileal mucosa.

Of the currently known strains of Lactobacillus, *Lactobacillus GG* (which is not yet available in India) meets all these criteria, however, its clinical efficacy is proven in only limited number of clinical situations (*vide infra*). In India, most of the preparations available are those of *Lactobacillus acidophiles* (Lactisyn, Lacktocil, Lactiflora) or *Lactobacillus sporogens* (Sporolin). Efficacy of none of these strains has been established in any substantial manner.

Situations in which certain probiotics have been shown to be useful

Lactobacillus GG has been shown to be somewhat effective in management of rotavirus diarrhea. In rota virus diarrhea, the average duration of diarrhea is reduced only by 18 hours or so, which may not be of much clinical benefit. It is not very effective in preventing *Clostridium difficile* (pseudomembranous colitis) diarrhea, or other bacterial diarrheas.

Sacchromyces boulardii has been effective in preventing travellers' diarrhea and diarrhea due to *Clostridium difficile*, but it has no role in all other types of diarrheas.

A combination of 3 probiotics (VSL # 3) including *Lactobacillus GG*, is likely to be introduced in the Indian market. Studies for its efficacy and safety are presently ongoing. It remains to be seen if it will be more effective than *Lactobacillus GG* in Rota virus diarrhea.

The practical implication of all this information is that while probiotics may be helpful in certain diarrheal situations, but we need much more information and evidence before they can be recommended in routine clinical practice. Also none of the available probiotic preparations have proven clinically useful till now. *Probably home made fresh curd/yoghurt is as good or better (as it also provides nutrition) as any of the available probiotic.*

Mucoid diarrhea

Non-invasive bacterial pathogens (like EPEC), parenteral infections, giardiasis etc. are the common causes of this type of diarrheal disease. Occasionally, this may occur in early stages of shigella infection. Vomiting is not a marked feature. Also dehydration, if at all present, is usually mild. These children also deserve a careful search for underlying parenteral infections and if present, treatment for the same. It may be prudent to obtain a routine stool examination to look for giardia, amoeba etc. and also for pus cells and red cells. If pus cells, more than 10 per H.P.F. or red cells are present, the child should be treated as invasive diarrhea (*vide infra*). Presence of giardial trophozoites would warrant treatment with metronidazole (20 mg/kg/day), otherwise these children also do not require any antibiotics or chemotherapeutic agents. If diarrhea does not subside in 3-5 days, repeat stool examination should be obtained.

Diarrhea with blood and mucus (invasive diarrhea) (Fig. 1.2)

This is now becoming a more frequent clinical problem. Typically children with invasive diarrhea (bacillary dysentery) present with frequent stools with blood and mucus, tenesmus and may be fever. The stools are usually small in amount and semiformed in consistency. The usual causative organisms are *Shigella, Salmonella, E.I.E.C.* (*Enteroinvasive Esch. Coli*) etc. As all of these organisms invade the colonic mucosa and multiply within the submucosa, they warrant absorbable, systemically effective, chemotherapeutic agents for their control and eradication. Drugs like nalidixic acid (55 mg/kg/day) furazolidone (7 mg/kg/day) or trimethoprim-sulfa (10 mg/kg/day of trimethoprim) are the drugs of choice. Chloramphenicol is too toxic for routine use and ampicillin is largely ineffective, as most of the gastrointestinal bacteria have developed resistance to this drug. As of today, nalidixic acid (55 mg/kg/day) is still the first choice antibiotic in children with bacillary dysentery.

With increasing resistance of shigella in certain parts of our country, other antibiotics, like 3rd generation cepholosparins (cefotaxime, ceftriaxone), fluoroquinolones (ciproflox, oflox etc.), and macrolid antibiotic like azithromycin may occasionally be required in individuals with shigella dysentery.

Only one drug should be given at a time and a minimum period of 2-3 days is required to get desirable response. First sign of clinical response is disappearance of blood from the stools. If this occurs, the drug should be continued for a total of 5 days and then stopped. Frequency of stools as also the passage of mucus may continue for 7-10 days and is not an indication for continuation or change of chemotherapeutic agent.

Value of stool cultures in deciding drug therapy

There is hardly any role of stool cultures in deciding drug therapy. In usual clinical situation, stool cultures give very little help in selecting drugs for children with acute diarrhea. If blood and mucus are present, child has to be treated on lines of invasive bacterial infection irrespective of the stool culture report and hence the culture is not required. Recent studies have clearly shown that presence of blood alone is the most useful indicator of antibiotic use in a child with acute diarrhea. In rest of the cases, stool cultures usually grow *Esch. coli* or *Klebsiella*. These organisms are even normally present in gastrointestinal tract and are not necessarily pathogenic. To define patho-genecity of *Esch. coli*, detailed toxigenic and tissue invasive studies are required, which are rarely available. In fact they are not even required as controlled trials have not shown any beneficial role of antibiotics even in proven enterotoxigenic *Esch. coli* diarrhea. Serotyping also is not usually available and even if available does not necessarily define the pathogenicity of isolated *Esch. coli*, as more and more untypable but pathogenic strains of *Esch. coli* are being identified. It is interesting to note that antibiotic sensitivity of isolated *Esch. coli* has no correlation with its pathogenicity and hence should not be made a basis for the choice of antibiotics.

Conclusions

It is apparent that a careful appraisal of clinical features like age of the child, consistency and content of stools, presence or absence of vomiting; coupled with detailed physical examination, can help in formulating rational drug therapy in majority of children with acute diarrhea. In doubtful cases, simple investigations like microscopic examination of stools and blood examination for total and differential cell count (and bandemia) may be obtained rather than using irrational drug therapy. Stool cultures have no value in routine practice. Remember, it is the cause of diarrhea which needs treatment, if any, rather than the diarrhea itself and in majority of the cases, the underlying cause (Rota, *ETEC, EPEC* etc.) is self limiting, requiring no treatment except replacement of fluids and electrolytes.

DIET IN DIARRHEA

No other aspect of diarrhea management has evoked as much controversy and as much diversity in practice as its dietary management. Classical treatise have suggested starvation for a variable period of 2-3 days and then gradual regrading of milk and other food. Many clinical and experimental observations which showed that stool volume increased on taking oral feeds, tended to substantiate this classical management. However, more recent studies have helped to rationalise the dietary management of children with acute diarrheal disease.

Frequent mention (in the western literature) of conditions like secondary lactose intolerance, cow's milk protein intolerance and other protein intolerances in association with diarrheal disease and increasing availability of cow's milk and lactose free substitutes, have further confused the practitioners with regard to the rational use of these therapeutic products. Before the current knowledge regarding dietary management is discussed it would be important to briefly review the background knowledge of pathogenetic factors operative in a diarrheal child which may have a bearing on the type of diet prescribed.

Diarrhea and Malnutrition

Each episode of diarrhea leads to compromise of nutritional status. Apart from active loss of nutrients, due to concomitant malabsorption, there is a variable intensity and duration of anorexia due to which the child's nutritional intake is compromised. If this is coupled with iatragenic starvation, the problem of nutritional deprivation may be further compounded. Thus, if not managed properly, each episode of diarrhea leads to a state of negative nitrogen balance and a variable period of growth failure. Repeated episodes may lead to occurrence of frank malnutrition. Malnutrition predisposes to an increased incidence, duration and severity of diarrhea. Mortality among severely malnourished children with diarrhea is almost 4 times than that in the normally nourished child. Thus diarrhea and malnutrition constitute a vicious cycle more so in (preschool age group) children living in tropical countries with poor environmental

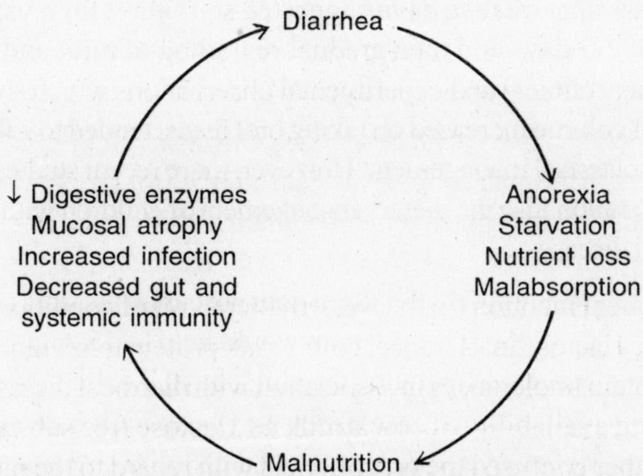

Fig. 2.1. Diarrhea and malnutrition : a vicious cycle.

hygiene. A proper dietary management during acute diarrhea, aimed at restoring normal nutritional status is thus of vital importance in breaking this vicious cycle. Dietary management is most crucial in ensuring not only successful outcome of the current episode but also in the prevention of future episodes.

Affect of nutritional intake on diarrheal disease

Earlier studies had noted increase in stool volume with increased food intake, leading to the practice of starving a child with diarrhea. In traditional systems of medicine also, diarrheal children have been variously starved. Nevertheless as long back as in 1948, Chang et al. demonstrated the benefit of early oral feeding in diarrheal cases. More recent, finely controlled, metabolic studies have also revealed that despite the presence of mild malabsorption (in children with diarrhea), the children who are given *ad libitum* food have a positive nitrogen balance and recover much faster with decreased duration of total diarrheal episode. It was realised that although these children are malabsorbing to some extent, but malabsorption occurs only for a fraction of the ingested food and the majority of food is anyway digested and absorbed, bringing the child in positive nutritional balance. It has been shown that 75 to 90% of ingested carbohydrates, fats and proteins in diet are absorbed even during acute diarrhea.

The development of glucose based O.R.S. and further modifications of it in the management of acute diarrhea, has further helped to clarify the dietary management of diarrheal children. Although glucose electrolyte based W.H.O. O.R.S. has been shown to be effective in correcting dehydration, it does not curtail the stool losses. The search for super O.R.S., which would help in decreasing the stool output besides rehydrating the child, has led to the discovery that substances like rice, lentils, barley etc. constitute a good substitute for glucose in O.R.S. The mean stool output and time to achieve rehydration is much shorter in diarrheal children fed on rice based

O.R.S. than those fed on glucose based W.H.O. O.R.S. In fact, various monosaccharides (glucose, fructose), disaccharides (sucrose), polysaccharides (starch), and amino acids (glycine, lysine etc.) can be used to promote solute-linked sodium and water absorption in acute diarrhea. Recently, even short- chain fatty acids have been shown to increase colonic absorption of water and electrolytes. Thus monosaccharides, disaccharides, short polymers of glucose, amino acids and short-chain fatty acids can all enhance water and electrolyte absorption. *A realisation that ordinary foods (like rice, khichri etc.), after all, consist of these substances only, has helped to suggest that **food is the best super O.R.S.*** Thus, if intake of water can be increased together with increased amounts of usually available foods in a mashed, easily digestible manner, the stool losses can be curtailed, hydration can be maintained and the nutritional status can be restored.

It has been shown that even during an acute diarrheal episode, more than 85% of dietary fats can be absorbed. Fats in the diet have the advantage that they increase the calorie content of food without increasing its bulk or its osmolarity. Thus, they are useful in making the so-called "Energy dense foods". It is important to use these foods during convalescence after an episode of diarrhea, to rapidly restore the nutritional balance. Their use would be even much more crucial if the child was already malnourished at the onset of diarrheal episode. Any of the vegetable oils or ghee can be added to *Dal, Khichri, Dalia* etc. in appropriate amounts, to make them more energy dense.

Cow's (or Bufallo's) milk in acute diarrhea

Some studies have shown that feeding of cow's milk during acute diarrheal stage may lead to development of cow's milk protein intolerance. This has been traced to increased permeability of gastrointestinal mucosa during diarrheal episode which permits absorption of macro molecules like milk proteins, with subsequent development of antibodies to milk proteins, which are able to perpetuate the intestinal mucosal damage and the episode of diarrhea. It has therefore been advised that "top" milk should be avoided during first 24 to 48 hours of diarrheal episode and regraded gradually thereafter.

This practice of avoidance and then regarding was universally practised till about 1980. However, several studies since then, have clearly shown that this is not at all necessary esp. in infants older than 6 months of age. These studies have shown that the average duration or persistence of diarrhea is not affected by continued "top" (Cow's, buffalo's, powdered) milk feeding in children with diarrhea.

In younger infants who are non breast fed and develop acute diarrhea, it will be prudent to stop milk feeds as long as the child is dehydrated. Thereafter, milk (undiluted) feeds can be restored in small quantities. To ensure adequate calories, it can be concentrated with cereals (rice, wheat, dalia) and with few drops of oil. Milk should not be diluted.

It must also be emphasised that "top" milk feeding in a non-breast-fed infant is the major source of high class (biological value) proteins which are so essential for achieving positive nitrogen balance and to maintain normal growth in infancy. Further "top" milk (as also breast milk) has 0.67 cal/ml, which is the most calorie dense food for infant, as most other infant foods (like *dalia*, *khichri*, mashed *dal* etc.) contain only 0.25 cal/ml when made in consistency suitable for infant feeding. Obviously to meet the calorie requirements, much smaller amounts of milk are required compared to other infant foods. Hence, as far as possible, milk (undiluted) feeding must continue in children with acute diarrhea. Incidence of milk protein intolerance, if any, is extremely small and should not deter us from continuing milk feeding in an infant.

Lactose intolerance and diarrheal disease

Occurrence of secondary lactose intolerance following a diarrheal episode was recognised as early as in 1965. The diagnosis can be easily confirmed by assessing the pH (< 5.5) and by testing for reducing substances in freshly passed stool water. The incidence is extremely low during acute diarrheal (< 5-7 days) illness. Even when present during acute diarrhea, lactose intolerance is usually mild (green/yellow reduction on Benedict's test) and transitory, not usually requiring withdrawl of milk. In any case, breast milk (which is much higher in lactose content) is usually well tolerated in acute diarrhea, even if biochemical evidence of lactose intolerance is present. Thus in most cases of acute diarrhea lactose (milk) withdrawl is not at all warranted.

On the other hand, evidence of lactose intolerance appearing for the first time after, or persisting beyond 5-7 days of the onset of diarrheal episode, usually suggests a persistent mucosal damage. The incidence of this late appearing lactose intolerance is not more than 3-5%. Even this is mostly transitory and quantitative (not all or none) in nature, requiring *reduction* and not withdrawl of dietary lactose and that too for not more than 5-7 days. (For details, see chapter on persistent diarrhea).

Micronutrients in diarrhea

Apart from providing adequate calories and proteins, it is also important to ensure adequate micronutrients in diet. In this regard two micronutrients are of special value.

Vitamin A is a vitamin which promotes mucosal integrity and may be helpful in decreasing diarrheal duration. However in controlled trials, vitamin A supplementation has not been helpful in decreasing diarrheal morbidity. But in a malnourished child, vitamin A levels may deplete rapidly during a diarrheal illness. This rapid depletion may even lead to keratomalacia within few hours leading to permanent blindness. Thus prompt vitamin A supplementation (1-2 laks I.M. *stat*) is very necessary in malnourished children with diarrhea or in children with prolonged diarrhea.

Zinc is another micronutrient which is widely distributed in body tissues and plays vital role in various matebolic processes as a part of various metallo-enzymes. Its deficiency, especially in tropical countries, is wide spread, being present in 30-40% of under 5 children. Zinc deficiency is associated with diarrheal prolongation, failure to thrive and even short stature.

Controlled trials have shown that zinc supplementation during acute diarrhea significantly shortens its duration and severity. Thus it is now recommended that zinc supplementation (10 mg/day for < 1 yr and 20 mg/day for > 1 yr old children) must be given to all children with acute diarrhea. The supplementation must continue for 14 days, as it helps to prevent future episodes of diarrhea (and also respiratory infections).

While the role of zinc supplementation is well demonstrated in comparatively malnourished children, a recent study from Turkey has shown this may not be of any benefit in normal nourished children.

A syndrome of metabolic disorder associated with zinc deficiency is described which results in severe prolonged watery diarrhea and acrodermatitis (Acrodermatitis enteropathica). Acrodermatitis is characterized by ulcerative/inflammatory lesions around the corners of the mouth and in the perianal area. In this condition high doses of zinc are required over a prolonged period.

Practical guidelines in planning dietary therapy

Following guidelines can be laid down in the dietary management of a diarrheal child based on our current understanding of underlying factors as listed above:

i) No child with acute diarrhea should be starved. Feeding should begin as soon as dehydration has been corrected.

ii) Breast feeding can and should be continued in all infants with diarrhea.

iii) Easily digestible soft food should be given *ad libitum* to the child as soon as, and as much as, he would like to have. Small frequent feeds would be preferable. Child should be encouraged to take *khichri*, *Dalia*, Mashed *bananas*, mashed *dal*, biscuits etc. The normal dietary intake should be restored as soon as possible.

iv) Rice based O.R.S. may be a better O.R.S. than glucose based O.R.S. as it would provide additional calories besides decreasing the stool volume. It should be supplemented with food as soon as possible.

v) In non breast fed infants below 6 months of age, amounts of top milk (cow's or buffalo's) should be reduced (not diluted) during first 24-48 hours of diarrheal episode and then increased gradually. Cereals like rice and small amounts of oil can be added to the top milk to increase energy density. This practice may be revised in view of ongoing research.

vi) It is not advisable to dilute milk during or after diarrheal episode. When lactose intolerance is proven, it may be alright to just restrict the total amount of milk (to about 30-50 ml/kg/day) and give remaining calories as cereals. This practice not only reduces the lactose load in the diet but also helps to maintain adequate calorie intake. Thus, this helps in quicker recovery from diarrheal episodes.

vii) Children recovering from a diarrheal episode need to have an extra intake to compensate for the nutrient deprivation. They may take as much as one and a half to two times their normal intake for upto 5-7 days after the episode of diarrhea and they should be encouraged to do so, even if the stools tend to become somewhat bulkier. Addition of vegetable oils to usual weaning foods would help in increasing the calorie content. This is even more important in malnourished children recovering from diarrhea.

viii) It is perfectly normal for an acute diarrheal episode to continue for 5-7 days. There is no need to start either milk substitutes or lactose free foods during this time i.e., there is no place for these foods in the management of acute diarrhea lasting for less than 7 days duration. Even after that, if the child is continuing to maintain hydration and nutritional status (weight gain appropriate for age) on normal food and fluids, there is no indication at all for substitution of milk foods, irrespective of stool fre-quency or consistency. Remember secondary lactose intolerance and cow's milk protein intolerance are both complicating factors responsible for protracted diarrhea, (diarrhea more than 14 days with weight loss) and are usually, not very significant pathogenetic factors in acute diarrhea. Also it would be well to remember that many milk substitutes (like soyabean milk) are more allergenic (35% Vs 2%) compared to cow's milk and hence introduction of these (soyabased) milks in a diarrheal child may predispose him to the development of soya protein intolerance and perpetuation of the diarrheal episode. Even if a low lactose or lactose-free diet is prescribed, soya-based feeds are better avoided. Home based foods like curd/*khichri* have proven to be better in controlling diarrhea and improving nutritional status. It provides both low lactose and probiotics (lactobacillus in curd), besides the desired nutrition.

ix) Indications for possible decrease in lactose contents of the ingested food exists only if diarrhea is prolonged beyond 7-14 days and lactose intolerance can be unequivocally demonstrated by stool examination. In our experience, associated systemic infections are more important in perpetuation of a diarrheal episode than any food intolerance (see Persistent diarrhea chapter).

x) All children with acute diarrhea should receive zinc supplementation for 14 days. This may be more crucial in malnourished children. Also all malnourished children with acute diarrhea should receive a stat dose of vitamin A (1-2 lakhs I.M.) to prevent keratomalacia.

ORAL AND INTRAVENOUS FLUID THERAPY IN DIARRHEA

In pediatric practice one is often confronted with disease states associated with significant fluid and electrolyte disturbances, requiring either oral or intravenous fluid therapy. Pediatric units at various medical colleges have evolved therapeutic regimes for different disease states which the residents learn by repetitious use without a basic understanding of biochemical disturbances. A wide variety of ready to use solutions with markedly different compositions are available in the market for therapeutic use and one is often handicapped in using these solutions rationally in the absence of this basic understanding. We shall here outline the rational use of oral and intravenous fluid therapy in pediatric practice with the background understanding of biochemical disturbances.

Oral Rehydration

Oral rehydration therapy (ORT) is now recognised as a powerful intervention in the treatment of dehydration due to acute diarrhea and has been described as "potentially the most important medical advance of the 20th century". ORT has been shown to be safe and efficacious and has now come to be recognised as the mainstay in the domicilliary management of diarrhea. The scientific basis of oral rehydration therapy arose from the fundamental observations that sodium transport across the intestinal mucosa, was enhanced by concurrent glucose transport. This *glucose linked sodium (and water) transport* is largely intact in diarrheas of varied etiologies and hence use of glucose-electrolyte solutions can help to prevent or correct dehydration in large majority of diarrheal episodes. Glucose in glucose-electrolyte solution can be replaced by any carbohydrate which is ultimately hydrolysed into glucose and absorbed as such. Both starch, present in various cereals (esp. rice), and sugar have been used successfully for rehydration in place of glucose. Certain amino-acids like glycine, lysine, etc. have also been found to enhance sodium and water absorption, just like glucose.

The World Health Organisation (W.H.O.) had earlier recommended an oral rehydration solution (ORS) containing 90 mEq of sodium and 110 mOsm of glucose per litre of solution together with citrate and potassium in appropriate amounts (Table 2.3). Although a lot of controversies surrounded its composition, particularly regarding its sodium content, yet it was used safely and effectively for oral rehydration in majority of patients if instructions regarding its use, as proposed by WHO, were followed strictly (*vide infra*).

Table 2.3, Composition of WHO, ORS (mOsm/litre)

	Original	*New hypo-osmolar*
Glucose	110	75
Na^+	90	75
K^+	20	20
Citrate	10	10
Total osmolarity	330	265

Hypo-osmolar ORS

The conventional WHO ORS has a total osmolarity of 330 mOsm/L. This is higher than that of plasma (i.e. 285 mOsm/L). Thus, WHO ORS withdraws water from intestinal surface into the lumen by its osmotic action, while at the same time glucose part of it helps to push sodium (and water) into the intestinal mucosa. Thus, while hydration is restored, yet the stool losses continue.

It has now been shown that solutions which are hypo-osmolar (200-265 mOsm/L) are better absorbed and help to decrease the stool losses significantly. Rice based ORS, besides providing calories, also help to decrease stool losses, as this is also hypo-osmolar in nature as the starch in rice gets hydrolysed into polymers of glucose, which, being large size particles, have much lower osmolarity.

Recently, WHO has suggested a revised formulation for its universal ORS. This ORS contains not only reduced sodium, but also has less osmolarity. This hypo-osmolar ORS has been shown to be more effective in not only restoring hydration but also in decreasing diarrheal losses by almost 20-30% and in better control of vomiting. Thus this ORS is better equipped to meet the parental demand of decreasing GI losses (diarrhea/vomiting) besides restoring hydration. This type of ORS is now gradually replacing the original WHO ORS in the Indian market and many new brands such as Rebalanz, Electrobion etc. are now available as hypoosmolar ORS. In fact this type of ORS will most likely replace conventional WHO ORS (with 90 mEq/L) or low sodium (Type B) ORS (with 60 mEq/L) available in the Indian markets till now.

Hypo-osmolar solution is not the same thing as low sodium solution. In the later, only the sodium content is lower than the WHO ORS while in the former, both the sodium and glucose contents have been readjusted to have a total decrease in osmolarity.

Fluids other than WHO O.R.S. can also be used for oral dehydration provided they contain a glucose substitute (to act as a substrate) and some electrolytes. Thus sugar salt solutions, rice water, dal water, coconut water etc. can also be used for oral rehydration therapy.

Oral rehydration therapy can be used for prevention and treatment of dehydration, and for maintenance of hydration in a diarrheal child. But conventional (high sodium) WHO solution by itself is not suitable for all these phases of hydration therapy. The fluids to be used during different phases of hydration therapy are detailed below :

i) *Prevention of dehydration:* Home available fluids like coconut water, barley water, *dal* water, Rice *Kanji*, etc.

should be used for this phase of hydration therapy. Alternatively low sodium glucose formulation or sugar-salt solution with four or five spoons of sugar and one teaspoon of salt to a litre of water (Sodium content 60 mEq/L) can be used. Fluids based on WHO formulations (containing 90 mEq/L of sodium) are not suitable for this phase of therapy.

ii) *Treatment of dehydration:* WHO type of ORS is to be used in calculated amounts (50 ml/kg and 100 ml/kg in 4 hours for mild and moderate dehydration respectively, or 75 ml/kg for "some dehydration", till dehydration is corrected. If the child is still dehydrated after 4 hours, then the same amounts of ORS may be repeated. This phase of rehydration would usually last 6-8 hours. If the child is still dehydrated after 8 hrs. then it would be preferable to use intra-venous therapy for some time. In infants < 3 months of age it would be preferable to use low sodium (50-60 mEq/L) containing ORS, even for this phase of rehydration. Hypo-osmolar ORS can probably be used as such in these infants also.

iii) *For maintenance of hydration:* As excess amounts of fluid losses usually continue even after correction of dehydration, it is important to continue giving extra fluids during this stage of hydration therapy also. However, the amounts of sodium losses in diarrheal stools in this phase of diarrhea is much less. Therefore, it is not advisable to continue the use of WHO formula alone during this period. It can be given with breast feeds (which contain only 4 mEq/Litre of sodium) or with feeds of plain water in 2 : 1 proportion. Alternatively oral rehydration solutions with sodium content of 50-60 mEq/litre or new hypo-osmolar ORS can be used safely. It is important to restore normal diet as soon as dehydration has been corrected.

Above mentioned guidelines for use of WHO ORS, in different phases of rehydration, were crucial when one was using conventional (original) WHO ORS. *Now with the availability of hypo-osmolar ORS, these guidelines may be less crucial and the current WHO ORS can probably be safely used in all phases of rehydration, without any modification.*

Apart from these general guidelines, which must be strictly adhered to, many other practical considerations need to be kept in mind while using ORT.

Preparing ORS

A variety of preparations are available in market (Table 2.4). They not only have different composition, on reconstitution, but also have different instructions for reconstitution. It is important, therefore, to carefully read the instructions for reconstitution and to familiarise

Table 2.4. Composition of Commercially available ORS

A) Glucose based

I. Hypo osmolar : Rebalanz, Walyte

II. Low Sodium
   - a) With Small Sachet for 200 ml & Large Sachet for 1000 ml
     Coslyte, Electral, Emlyte S
   - b) With only one large sachet for 1000 ml
     Dextrolyte, Leclyte
   - c) Available as ready to drink fluids
     Orolyte P.

III. High Sodium (Na^+ 90 mOsm, Osmolarity 330 mOsm/L)
   - a) With small Sachet for 200 ml & large sachet for 1000 ml
     Electrobion, Emlyte, Peditral
   - b) With only Large Sachet for 1000 ml
     Electrolac, Infalyte, Oral N.E.P.C., Prolyte Punarjal, Relyte, Quicksol

B. Rice based ORS (Na^+ 90, Osmolarity 220 mOSm/L) – now getting replaced
   Cerelyte, Ricetral

C. Super ORS. Dextrose-Glycine based (Na^+ 90, Osmolarity 442 mOsm/L) Speed oral (Glucose 20 gm%, Glycine 22.0%)

oneself with the composition of 1 or 2 types of ORS. Currently the ORS packets are available either in one large sachet (which is to be dissolved in 1 litre of water) or as 5 small sachets within one large sachet. Each of the small sachet is to be dissolved in 200 ml (1 glass) of water. It is important to measure the amounts of water carefully as household measures are seldom standardized.

There is no need to boil water for preparing ORS. The ORS should be used within 12-24 hours of its preparation, otherwise it can get contaminated. Physician should prescribe only that brand about whose composition and method of preparation he is absolutely certain. Parents should always be advised that if the prescribed brand is not available then they should bring back the dispensed pack to the physician for clear instructions.

Inadequate intake of ORS by newborn and infants is an important cause of treatment failure and may even be fatal. Thus it is very important to advise parents about the correct amounts of ORS to be administered. While for correcting dehydration 75 ml/kg of ORS should be given over 4 hours, for prevention of dehydration at least 100 ml (200 ml for > 1 year old) of ORS should be given for each loose stool. Oral rehydration for dehydrated children must be done under close supervision with monitoring of intake, stool frequency, urine output, vomiting etc. If dehydration is not corrected within 6-8 hours or if it worsens, intravenous hydration should be given.

Types of ORS

Hypo-osmolar ORS, with a decreased sodium and glucose content and lower osmolarity can probably be used safely and effectively in all children irrespective of the cause of diarrhea. The other available oral rehydration solutions can be broadly categorized in those containing high sodium of 90 mEq/litre and those containing low sodium 50-60 mEq/litre (Table 2.4). Which one to use? The solutions containing 50-60 mEq/litre of sodium are safe and efficacious for prevention and maintenance phase and as 90% of diarrheal episodes in the community are not associated with dehydration, this type of solutions would be suitable in majority of cases. These solutions would probably be also ideal for rehydration of neonates and young infants (< 3 months old) because of the limited sodium handling capacity at this age. Also, most diarrheal episodes are due to either rotavirus or non-toxigenic bacteria and in them the stool sodium losses are low (< 50 mEq/litre). Therefore, in these cases also, ideal rehydration solution would be a low sodium containing ORS only.

For older children especially with toxigenic (cholera like) diarrhea, conventional WHO type of solutions (Na 90) are preferable for rehydration. In actual clinical practice therefore, WHO type of oral rehydration solution is appropriate for a very small minority of diarrheal episodes and for a limited phase of hydration (i.e. correction of deficit in a cholera like watery diarrhea). In large majority of diarrheal episodes, low sodium ORS are more physiological and appropriate.

Home made ORS

Oral rehydration solution can also be made with sugar and salt available at home. For this purpose one should add one teaspoon of sugar and one, 2 finger pinch of salt to one glass (200 ml) of water. A bit of lemon juice can be added which not only enhances the taste but also provides some citrate and some potassium. In this solution sugar (sucrose) provides the necessary solute for the transport of sodium and water. This home made ORS has the advantage of being readily and cheaply available and more acceptable, however, as large number of errors can occur in making the home made ORS (sugar and salt content interchanged with disasterous results), therefore, its use has been abandoned in public health programmes.

Super ORS and Rice ORS

Failure to control the symptoms of diarrhea with the use of glucose/sucrose electrolyte solutions, has led to the search of other solutions which may help in curbing the stool losses and thus in providing symptomatic relief, apart from maintaining hydration. Starch (Rice-electrolyte solution) or Glycine based ORS have been found to be useful in some studies and are referred to as super ORS. However, the reductions in diarrheal stools obtained, even with the use of these so-called super ORS, has not been very significant and definitely not consistent with marked increase (about 3 to 4 fold) in the cost of oral rehydration therapy with the use of these super ORS esp. those containing glycine. Recent studies have established that glycine really has hardly any usefulness as a super ORS.

Among super ORS, Rice based ORS (50 gm puffed rice cooked in 1 litre of water, with one spoon of salt) has proved to be most efficacious. This is now freely available in Indian markets, as ready to mix solutions (Ricetral). Starch present in rice gets broken into monosaccharide and oligo polysaccharides which promote the sodium and water transport across the intestine. Overall osmolarity of rice ORS is less than conventional ORS and this may be the reason for its better efficacy.

However, rice based ORS, made from processed rice based infant foods (e.g. nestum), is not as effective as puffed rice based rice ORS.

ORS in a Child with Vomiting

Vomiting *per se* is not a contraindication to oral rehydration therapy. Given in small amounts with spoon and cup, ORT can help in control of vomiting and has been used successfully for rehydration in such children also. One or two vomitings despite use of ORS, should not be a cause of concern but if the vomitings are profuse or persistent, then obviously the ORT must be abandoned in favour of intravenous therapy. Vomiting are much less with the use of hypoosmolar ORS.

ORT and Control of Diarrhea

While ORT is quite successful in achieving rehydration, unfortunately it does not control the problem of diarrhea. The stool losses continue as before or may even increase. This is often frustrating to the physicians and exasperating to the parents and is one of the major obstacles against general acceptance of oral rehydration therapy. A thorough understanding of this by physicians and explanation to the parents "*that diarrhea itself will take 3-5 days to settle, while ORT would largely prevent dehydration and hospitalisation*", usually helps in building the confidence of parents. A suggestion to the parents that diarrhea is really an attempt by the body to "*flush out the toxins" and by itself is not bad, as long as enough fluids can replace the flushed out fluids*", can often help them to understand and make them less insistent on controlling diarrhea as such. As pointed above, hypoosmolar ORS (including Rice based ORS) can help to decrease the purge rate.

When should ORT be terminated?

Oral rehydration therapy should be terminated:

i) As soon as abnormal losses of diarrheal stool are under control.

ii) If the vomiting is persistent and the child is unable to retain the oral rehydration fluids.

iii) If the dehydration is moderately severe or if it worsens on ORT. In this regard failure to establish adequate urination within 6-8 hours of ORT should be considered as an important indication for use of intravenous fluids.

iv) Complications like abdominal distension and convulsions develop.

v) ORT is usually unsuccessful in following conditions and should be replaced by intravenous fluids.

a) Very high purge rate (> 10 ml/kg/hr stool fluid losses)
b) Persistent vomitings
c) Severe acidosis/Severe dehydration
d) Convulsions/Abdominal distension
e) Septicemic illness
f) Glucose-Galactose intolerance (rare)
g) Severe dyselectrolytemia (occasional success stories of ORS not withstanding)

ORT in Newborns

Diarrhea in newborns largely occurs in two diverse clinical settings. One, in which a normal breast fed baby has an increased frequency and liquidity of stools (normal, increased frequency) and the other, in which diarrhea is due to a systemic bacterial illness like septicemia, meningitis etc. Use of ORT in either of these situations is absolutely unwarranted as, in the first instance, it is not required (and may lead to abnormal sodium and water retention) and in the second instance, immediate hospitalisation and management with intravenous fluids and antibiotics is mandatory. Delays in hospitalisation because of the temptation to use ORT at home can be catastrophic in these situations. *Thus, by and large ORT in newborns in domicillary settings cannot be justified.*

In highly controlled and supervised situations (in a hospitalised newborn), ORT has been shown to be effective in newborns also, but use of conventional WHO type of ORS, without additional water can lead to hypernatremia and excess retention of water in upto 25% of neonates. ORT can be even more dangerous in a baby receiving simultaneous "top" (cow's milk) feeds, which also have high (27 mEq/L) sodium content. It is better to use low sodium

ORS in young infants. There have been no trials yet to prove the safety of new hypo-osmolar ORS in neonates.

ORT in conditions other than diarrhea and vomiting

There is an increasing tendency to use ORT for conditions other than diarrhea and vomiting. Sometimes it is being used even as a health and restorative drink. A company has come out with a solution containing huge amounts of glucose together with the electrolytes and is propagating it as a health drink. It is to be remembered that ORT enhances not only water absorption but also sodium absorption and if it is used in conditions not associated with excessive sodium and water losses, it can cause dangerous hypernatremia. Also, large concentrations of glucose (> 3%) can lead to osmotic diarrhea and also to marked enhancement of sodium absorption and occurrence of hypernatremia. *Glucose-electrolyte solutions have a definite pathophysiological role and they must not be used in place of plain glucose feeds, or in non- diarrheal conditions.*

Intravenous fluid therapy

Intravenous fluid therapy is the mainstay of treatment in a wide variety of conditions of childhood. Apart from diarrhea and dehydration, it is often used as a maintenance therapy and to deliver high doses of antibiotics for conditions like pneumonia and meningitis. It is very important to deliver the right amounts of fluid at the appropriate rate of infusion while using the intravenous route, otherwise dangerous overhydration can develop rapidly. For practising intravenous fluid therapy in a rational manner it is important to understand the maintenance and deficit requirements of fluids and electrolytes as also the composition of various, ready to use, solutions available in the market.

Maintenance Requirements

Although fluid requirements can more scientifically be calculated on the basis of body surface area or on the basis of caloric expenditure, in clinical practice the method often used is that based on age and body weight because these parameters are readily available (Table 2.5). It is important to weigh the child accurately (with least clothing) to avoid wrong calculations.

Table 2.5. Maintenance Fluid Requirements

Age	*Fluid ml/kg/ 24 hr*	*Age*	*Fluid ml/kg/ 24 hr*
7 days - 3 mth	150	1-3 yrs	100
3-6 mth	130	3-7 yrs	80
6 mth-1 yr	120	> 7 yrs	60

Electrolyte Requirements

Maintenance requirement of sodium and potassium can also be calculated on the basis of body weight or surface area, but in practice it is best to calculate on the basis of *per litre of infusion fluids* being used (Table 2.6). This method also constantly reminds us that fluids in children must be given in a uniform manner i.e. every bottle of fluid must contain 30-40 mEq/litre of sodium (that is one part of normal saline and 3 parts of glucose) unlike adults where one can safely use 3 bottles of glucose followed by one bottle of saline over a 24 hours period. Also potassium concentration in infusion fluids should not exceed 20 mEq/litre for maintenance purposes.

Table 2.6. Maintenance Requirements of Electrolytes as mEq/litre of infusion fluids

Age	*Sodium*	*Potassium*
> 3 months	30-40	20
< 3 months	20-30	20

Thus solutions containing about 40 mEq/litre of sodium and 20 mEq/litre of potassium (Isolyte M) are quite suitable for maintenance purposes. In young children (< 3 months of age) solutions containing 20-30 mEq/litre of sodium (Isolyte P) are alright for maintenance purposes. The requirements of sodium for young infants is less because they have low renal concentration capacity. If excess amounts of sodium are given at this age, sodium and water retention can occur in the body, which may be quite dangerous. As normal saline contains about 155 mEq/L of sodium, maintenance requirements can be calculated as N/4 (>3 months of age) or N/6 saline (<3 months of age).

Maintenance requirements of other electrolytes

For short term use (2-3 days), it is not so important to give maintenance requirements of other electrolytes like calcium, phosphates, bicarbonate etc., because they are required in extremely small amounts. Their addition in routine maintenance fluids for short term only becomes a source of confusion and errors. It further serves to increase the cost of intravenous fluids.

Intravenous solutions available commercially

Most available solutions for intravenous use, mention the composition of various electrolytes in term of mEq/litre (Table 2.7) Some of the solutions may only mention the contents of various electrolytes as gms/litre. In that case one can calculate the amounts in mEq/litre by the formula :

$$\text{mEq/L} = \frac{\text{Gms/litre}}{\text{Gm. mol.}} \times 1000$$

(Gm mol. of any salt is its molecular weight expressed in grams). The Gm mol of some commonly used salts are given in Table 2.8,

e.g, 0.9% (normal saline) will contain $\frac{9}{58.5} \times 1000 = 155$

mEq/litre of sodium and 155 mEq/litre of chloride.

Table 2.7. Composition of Available I.V. Fluids

S. No.	I.V. Fluid	Dextrose mOsm/L	Na (mEq/L)	K (mEq/L)	Cl (mEq/L)	Bicarb	Total (mOsm/L)
1.	5% Dextrose	277	–	–	–	–	277
2.	10% Dextrose	555	–	–	–	–	555
3.	Isotonic Saline	–	155	–	155	–	310
4.	5% D.N.S.	277	154	–	154	–	585
5.	Dextrose Saline (5% Dextrose, 0.9% Saline)	277	77	–	77	–	431
6.	*N/4 Glucose Saline (3 parts 5% Dextrose, 1 part Isotonic Saline)	207	37.5	–	37.5	–	–
7.	*N/4 Glucose Saline with 15% Kcl 1 ml/100 ml	207	37.5	20	57.5	–	–
8.	Ringer Lactate	–	131	5	111	29	–
9.	Multiple electro-lyte Electrolyte G Leclyte G/PDlyte G	277	69	13	146	65	571
10.	Multiple electro-lyte P Electrolyte P/ Kidral/Leclyte P/PP lyte P	(Maintenance I.V. Solution for infants < 6 months) 277	38.5	17	19	36.5	398
11.	Multiple electro-lyte E. Electrolyte/ Leclyte E PD Lyte	277	160	10	103	5	633
12.	Electrolyte M Leclyte M/Leclyte	277	55.0	35	37	–	457
13.	Electrolyte (R) Leclyte R	277	58	16	44	–	449

* Reconstituted in wards for day-to-day purpose.

Table 2.8. Gm. mol of some commonly used salts

Salt	*Gm. mol.*	*Usually available as*
Sodium chloride (Na(23) Cl(35.5)	58.5	Isotonic saline (0.9% solution) containing 155 mEq/litre
Potassium chloride (Kcl) K (39), cl (35.5)	74.5	15% solution containing 1 mEq/ml
Sodium Bicarbonate ($NaHCO_3$) Na(23) HCO_3 (1+ 12+48)	84	7.5% solution containing 0.9 mEq/ml
Calcium chloride ($CaCl_2$) Ca(40) Cl_2(71)	55.5 *	10% solution containing 180 mEq/litre calcium

* Bivalent

Deficit therapy

Deficit therapy is most frequently required for dehydration produced by diarrheal disease. Here losses of both fluid and electrolytes are occurring. The severity of dehydration can be assessed by clinical examination and history following standard criteria (see Table 1.3 in overview of acute diarrhea).

Deficit fluid requirements can then be assessed by the degree of dehydration. *It is usually endeavoured to correct dehydration in first eight hours of fluid therapy and the fluids to be administered during this time should contain both the deficit fluids as well as the maintenance fluids required for this eight hour period.* Body weight deficit, maintenance and total fluids required in first eight hours of admission in various grades of dehydration are given in Table 2.9.

It should be noted that while doing deficit correction we are not replacing the total deficit but only about half of the deficit and we allow the rest of deficit to be taken care of by body's own homeostatic mechanisms over a period of time. The same principle (i.e. of under correction) applies to deficit of various electrolytes like sodium, bicarbonate, potassium etc.

Table 2.9. Deficit Fluid Therapy (ml/kg)

Average degree of dehydration	*Body Wt. deficit*	*Deficit fluid (ml/kg)*	*Deficit replacement in 8 hrs.*	*1/3rd* maintenance*	*Total fluid in first 8 hrs.*
Mild	3-5%	30-50	Nil	50	50
Moderate	7-10%	70-100	50	50	100
Severe	10-15%	120-150	100	50	150

* 7 days - 3 years of age.

* The amounts are decreased thereafter as per maintenance requirements (See Table 2.6).

As the amounts of sodium losses are also much more in vomitus and diarrheal stools (Table 2.10), during deficit therapy we try to give more sodium also. Thus instead of giving a solution containing 30-40 mEq/litre of sodium, we give solutions containing 70-75 mEq/litre (half strength isotonic saline or 0.45% saline). In older children (above 6 years of age) especially with severe degree of dehydration, the deficit correction may be done even with solutions containing 140-150 mEq/litre of sodium (Isotonic (0.9%) saline or Ringer's lactate).

Table 2.10. Estimation of concurrent losses of electrolytes (mEq/Litre)

	Sodium	*Potassium*	*Chloride*	*Bicarb*
Vomiting (or gastric aspirate)	90	20	110	–
Diarrheas*	30-60	20	70	5-10**
Cholera	90-110	20	110	20

NB : These are approximate values. Electrolytes should be monitored and appropriately replaced whenever prolonged losses occur.

* Vary with severity of diarrhea (high sodium with high purge rate).

** With toxigenic diarrheas.

If the child is dehydrated, his urine output is likely to be low. As long as adequate renal function is not established body is accumulating potassium, *hence no potassium should be added in the infusion fluids unless adequate urination is established.*

Deficit therapy in older children

As maintenance fluid requirements in children above 3 years of age (in ml/kg) are low, appropriate corrections have to be made for them while giving deficit therapy. Thus in a 6-8 years old child, 8 hours maintenance is only 20 ml/kg, this added with deficit requirements in mild, moderate or severe dehydration will give the total requirements for 8 hrs. of deficit fluid therapy as 20, 80 and 120 ml/kg respectively in 8 hours (Ref. Table 2.10), instead of 50, 100 and 150 ml in younger children and infants.

Calculating drip rate

With usual drip sets, each ml of solution has 15 drops. The drip rate with these type of drip sets can be calculated by the formula :

As many 100 ml/24 hrs — As many drops/minute

If a child has to get 400 ml in 8 hrs, i.e. 1200 ml in 24 hrs, then his drip rate should be adjusted to 12 drops/minute (for 8 hrs). This will ensure administration of 400 ml fluid in 8 hrs.

In infant burrette sets, the drop size is smaller and 1 ml contains 60 drops. Appropriate corrections will have to be made for the drip rate.

Of course now a days, infusion pumps are available which can be adjusted to deliver the required amounts of fluids in designated time.

WHO protocol for intravenous fluids

Recent regime for intravenous rehydration being propagated by

WHO sponsored protocols, recommends using Ringer's lactate for all children irrespective of age. However, it must be remembered that *WHO protocols recommend intravenous fluids only for correction of severe rehydration (i.e. with peripheral circulatory failure)* and that too only till the peripheral circulatory failure is corrected. Thus it recommends only 30-50 ml/kg of Ringer's Lactate in about 2 hours time and then to continue rehydration with ORS. *Ringer's lactate is not recommended for total correction of fluid deficit or for milder degrees of dehydration.* What we are writing here is about the use of intravenous fluid therapy for any degree of dehydration which may occasionally be required even with less than severe dehydration, if the child is vomiting or has complications like abdominal distension etc. Using Ringer lactate in children with no dehydration or with mild/moderate dehydration can cause severe hypernatremia.

Bicarbonate or Lactate in Deficit Therapy

Successful rehydration can be achieved in majority of children with just 0.45% saline in 5% dextrose, calculated according to the degree of dehydration, but if the dehydration is severe, or if clinical signs of acidosis (deep and fast breathing) are present, then it may be wise to include bicarbonate or lactate also in the deficit fluid therapy. After taking blood samples for sodium, potassium, bicarbonate and pCO_2. (If facilities are available), soda bicarb (3 mEq/kg or 3-5 ml/kg of 7.5% solution) can be added to the deficit fluid. This is a concentrated solution (containing 900 mEq/L of HCO_3^-) and hence should always be diluted with at least 5 parts of dextrose. This 1/6th diluted solution of 7.5% soda bicarb contains sodium and bicarbonate in concentrations of 150 mEq/litre each and is isotonic with plasma. 20 ml/kg of this 1/6th diluted 7.5% soda bicarbonate solution can be given over 1 hour to correct acidosis. It elevates plasma bicarbonate levels by just 5-8 mEq/litres.

If plasma HCO_3^- levels are available then amount of bicarbonate required can be calculated by the formula :

$(28 - \text{Observed } HCO_3) \times \text{wt in kg} \times 0.5$

This gives the total deficit. Normally we endeavour to correct only half of this deficit.

Example : A one year old child weighing 8 kg is clinically acidotic. His plasma bicarbonate is 10 mEq/L. Calculate the amounts of bicarb required for this child.

Calculation :

Bicarb deficit is $(28 - 10) \times 8 \times 0.5 = 72$ mEq/L

We need to correct half (i.e. 36 mEq/L) of this.

Thus he will require 40 ml of 7.5% Sodium bicarb, which mean 5 ml/kg. This will need to be made as 1/6th solution. Thus he will require 40 ml of 7.5% Sodium bicarbonate and 200 ml of 5% Dextrose. Thus 240 ml solution can be given our 1 to 2 hours. This will also meet his Sodium and fluid requirements over this period.

Ringer's lactate could also be used for correction of acidosis and fluid deficit. However, lactate in Ringer's solution is converted to bicarbonate in the liver and hence caution is to be exercised, if it is used in a child with compromised liver function.

Management of severe dehydration with or without peripheral circulatory failure (Fig. 2.2)

In severe dehydration, at least one half of the calculated deficit should be given in first two hours. This rapid initial infusion is done in an attempt to restore renal blood flow and to re-establish urination at the earliest because prolonged reduction in renal blood flow may lead to acute tubular necrosis (ATN) and acute renal failure (ARF). It is also prudent to use Ringer's lactate or normal saline at least till urination is established.

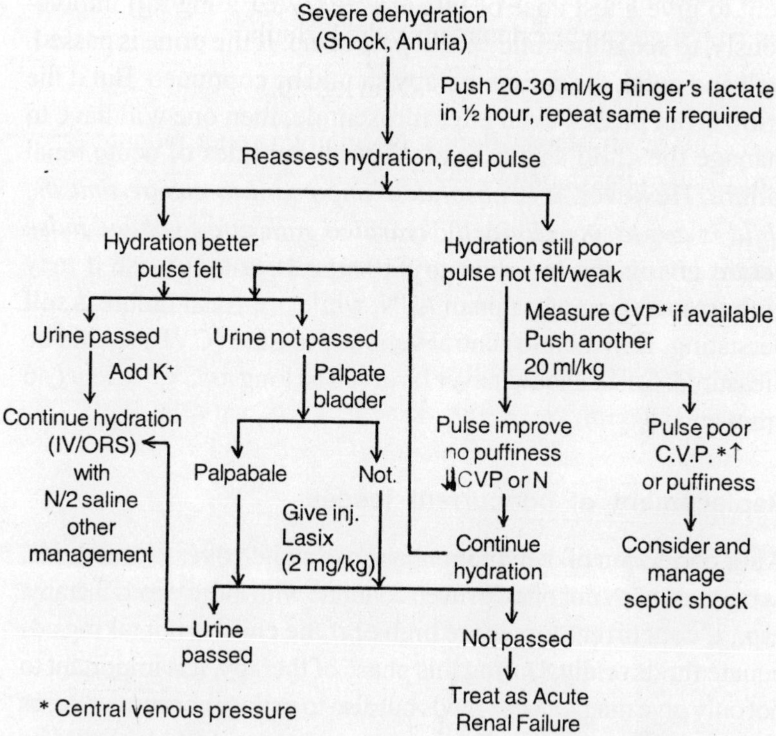

Fig. 2.2. Management algorithm for severe dehydration.

When the child presents initially to us with severe dehydration and anuria, it is assumed that anuria is prerenal due to plasma volume depletion and decreased renal blood flow, and an attempt is made to restore the plasma volume rapidly. Initial attempt should be to establish a good peripheral venous access and to give at least 20 ml/kg fluids as bolus. Fluids to be given are either Ringer's lactate or isotonic saline. No potassium is given till adequate urination is established. In situations where a peripheral venous canulation is difficult, intra-osseous fluids can be given to replenish the vascular volume rapidly. However, if after 1 to 2 hours, during which time at least 40-50 ml/kg of fluid have been pushed, the child looks hydrated with good pulse but does not pass urine, then we must seriously suspect the possibility of ATN. At this stage it would be prudent to give a test dose of furosemide (*Lasix* 2 mg/kg) intravenously, to see if the child would pass urine. If the urine is passed, well and good, the deficit therapy should be continued. But if the urine is not passed even after furosemide, then one will have to manage the child as a case of ATN on the lines of acute renal failure. However, *it is absolutely important to ensure that the child is appearing clinically hydrated with good volume pulse before giving the test dose of furosemide* as otherwise it may give erroneous impression of ATN, while pre-renal failure is still persisting. If available central venous pressure (CVP) should be measured. Lasix should never be given as long as CVP is low (<6 cm/water).

Replacement of concurrent losses

After correction of dehydration, one can switch over to oral fluids, as outlined above or one can even continue with intravenous therapy, esp., if concurrent losses are high or if the child is not taking adequate fluids orally. During this phase of therapy, it is important to not only give maintenance fluids but also to replace concurrent losses in appropriate amounts. The concurrent losses of fluids should be estimated as nearly as possible by close clinical observations and/or by actual measurements. The amounts of electrolytes lost in them can then be assessed by knowing the electrolyte content in gastric aspirate or lower intestinal losses (Table 2.10). The replacement should then be done with appropriately constituted fluids. Serum electrolytes must be monitored periodically and adjustments in fluid composition made accordingly.

Isotonic dehydration

Most often dehydration in acute diarrhea is isotonic or isonatremic, that is, there are proportionate losses of water and sodium in stools and the serum sodium remains between 130 to 145 mEq/litre. The management outlined above is usually adequate.

Hyponatremic dehydration

Loss of excess amounts of sodium compared to water loss, or replacement of fluid losses with plain water may result in hyponatremic dehydration. Apart from the signs and symptoms seen in isonatremic dehydration, these children may have drowsiness, lethargy and convulsions. Clinically, the child appears much more dehydrated than the actual fluid losses during diarrhea. Oliguria is even more marked in these children.

Large majority of cases of hyponatremic dehydration can be managed on the lines mentioned above for isonatremic dehydration. However, if the serum sodium is less than 120 mEq/litre and is accompanied with symptoms like convulsions, a rapid correction of serum sodium may be required. *In actual clinical practice, however, it is rarely required.* If sodium levels are known, then the amount of sodium required can be calculated by the formula

(135-observed Serum Sodium) × wt. in kg × 0.6.

This will give the total sodium deficit but we normally give only half of this rapidly so as to raise the sodium levels to 125-126. It is worthwhile to remember that the total deficit correction, together with 24 hrs. maintenance requirement, should be given over 24 hours rather than 8 hours.

Example : Hyponatremic dehydration

A one year old infant with acute diarrhea and vomiting has been brought in with convulsions for last 10 minutes. He is moderately dehydrated and weighs 8.0 kg. His serum sodium is 118 mEq/L. Calculate the fluid/electrolyte therapy.

Fluid required in 1st 8 hours :

Moderate dehydration 100 ml/kg = 800 ml

in next 16 hours (2/3rd of maintenance)

100 ml/kg = 800 ml

Sodium required :

Deficits $(135 - 118) \times 0.6 \times 8 \quad = \quad 17 \times 0.6 \times 8$

$= \quad 82$ mEq.

Maintenance for 24 hours $= 8 \times 3 \quad = \quad 24$ mEq

Total sodium required in 24 hrs. $\quad = \quad 106$ mEq in

Half of sodium (50 mEq) is given rapidly as 300 ml normal saline in 2 hours and then 500 ml N/2 solution in 6 hours and then 800 ml N/5 solution in next 16 hours, as given below.

	Fluid	*Na^+*
1st 2 hours	300 ml normal saline*	50 mEq
Next 6 hours	500 ml N/2 saline	37.5 mEq
Next 16 hours	800 ml N/4 saline	20 mEq
Total fluid (24 hrs)	1600 ml	107.5 mEq

* Or Ringer Lactate

More commonly, hyponatremia occurs without dehydration (dilutional hyponatremia) e.g. in acute renal failure and in inappropriate ADH secretion etc. In these cases the management consists in restricting fluids (less than 2/3rd of maintenance) rather than giving more sodium.

In malnourished children the serum sodium is often low (< 130 mEq/litre). This is usually asymptomatic and no attempt should be made to correct this "hyponatremia" by giving high sodium fluids, as the total body sodium is already high in malnourished children despite low serum sodium.

Hypernatremic Dehydration

As such hypernatremic dehydration is rare in our clinical practice. However, it could occur in formula fed neonates and infants given ORS or if errors in mixing ORS occur. One of the cases of hypernatremia we had seen had occurred in an infant being given ORS in concentration of one teaspoon to one ounce of water (like powder milk feeds)!

Hypernatremic dehydration is an extremely dangerous situation resulting in high mortality and frequent sequelae among survivors. Because of the maintenance of plasma volume, at the cost of intracellular fluid deprivation, classical signs of dehydration like loss of skin turgor and depression of fontanelle, oliguria etc. are absent in these cases and child may look deceptively well. Only thing discernible at this stage may be just an anxious look. Then the child develops symptoms like shrill cry, neck retraction and convulsions. Later still, he may go into shock. It is very important to suspect this diagnosis early. *Well-nourished top-fed infants who look apparently well hydrated despite large diarrheal losses*, are the prime suspects for this condition.

Management : Serum electrolytes, plasma bicarbonate and blood urea should be obtained. If shock is present it should be managed with either Ringer's lactate or plasma infusion. Once the shock is corrected then solution containing 50-60 mEq/litre of sodium should be infused at a rate of 70-80 ml/kg/day. Total fluids are restricted because ECF volume is usually well maintained and the sodium solution of 50-60 mEq/L is given to ensure gradual reduction of serum sodium. Total correction should be accomplished slowly, over 48 hours period. Repeated clinical and biochemical monitoring is essential to achieve a favourable outcome.

Hypokalemia

Serum potassium levels less than 3.5 mEq/litre may be seen frequently in dehydrated children particularly those having malnutrition. Intravenous infusion with maintenance potassium (20 mEq/litre) together with early restoration of oral feeding (including fruit juice etc.) is usually effective and safe. When oral feeding cannot be restored early, because of either abdominal distension or vomiting, then one may increase the infusion rate to 30 mEq/litre. *Potassium should never be given as a straight injection or in concentrations greater than 30-40 mEq/litre of the infusion fluids, as higher concentrations can be immediately fatal.* Periodic monitoring of serum potassium and also of the ECG (if available) should be obtained to adjust the therapy.

3

Prolonged Diarrhea

DEFINITIONS

Various terminologies have been used to define those cases who have diarrhea over a long period of time. Thus, terms like persistent, protracted, intractable, recurrent, chronic, chronic malnourishing etc. have been used to describe diarrheal episodes of longer duration. These terms have been used interchangeably and to describe children with apparently different clinical syndromes. Some of them consider malabsorption syndromes as synonymous with chronic diarrhea. Thus, for an ordinary practitioner it becomes extremely difficult to develop a clinical approach to a child with so-called chronic diarrhea.

To our mind, children presenting with diarrhea over a long period of time (prolonged diarrhea) fall under three clinically distinct clinical syndromes each one of which represents different etiopathogenesis and require a different line of management. These syndromes are :

Persistent diarrhea : This has been defined by WHO as a diarrheal illness (passage of 3 or more loose stools) of presumed infectious etiology, starting acutely and lasting for more than 14 days. This syndrome is largely seen in infancy with more than 60%

episodes occurring in infants < 6 months of age and 90% before 1 year of age. Although not all of these children warrant active therapeutic intervention, but from an epidemiological viewpoint it is an extremely useful definition, as it helps to delineate those episodes which require more careful attention. This can be easily applied in the field by health workers also. 3 to 20% of acute diarrheal episodes (average 10%) tend to become persistent. Within this group two more terminologies are often used.

Protracted diarrhea : Persistent diarrhea episodes which are associated with failure to thrive have been labelled as protracted diarrhea. Although the word "protracted" only implies prolongation or drawn out, yet it is preferable to use this term only for those episodes of persistent diarrhea which get complicated with weight loss. Some authorities have also called these episodes as chronic malnourishing diarrhea. From clinical point of view this is the most useful definition as it helps to pin point those very children who are at an increased risk of dying because of prolonged diarrhea and hence always require active therapeutic intervention. Weight loss or inadequate weight gain in a diarrheal episode, may begin as early as 7-10 days but usually does not occur before 2 to 3 weeks of the onset of the diarrheal episode. Only 10% of persistent diarrheal episodes develop the problem of weight loss or inadequate weight gain.

Intractable diarrhea : Avery et al. (1977) defined a group of young infants (< 3 months of age) who had prolonged watery diarrhea and in whom repeated stool cultures (at least 3) were negative for all known enteropathogens. They labelled them as suffering from "intractable" (non-diagnosible and unmanageable) diarrhea. These infants had a very high mortality. However, this term is not used much now-a-days as similar clinical picture (as described by Avery et al.) can be seen even in infants upto 2 to 3 years of age and is not limited to young infants only. Further with identification of several new enteropathogens, it is difficult, if not impossible to process even one stool sample for all known enteropathogens. Also this definition is probably unsuitable because of its undue emphasis on enteropathogens as causative factor of persistent diarrhea, while really speaking multiple factors are operative in the causation and perpetuation of persistent diarrheal episodes. In any case, now-a-days most of the persistent diarrheal episodes can not only be managed but can possibly be even prevented and hence use of term "intractable" is largely unwarranted.

Recurrent diarrhea : Here the child (mostly between 6 months to 5 years of age) suffers from recurrent but distinct episodes of acute diarrhea. Even normally, an average preschool child in India and other tropical countries gets about 2-3 episodes per year and in urban slum areas this may be as much as 6-8 episodes per year.

There is no unanimity as to how many episodes of diarrhea in a year constitute recurrent diarrhea. However, in general, occurrence of 6 or more episodes per year could be defined as recurrent diarrhea. By the same token more than 3 episodes in 6 months or 2 or more episodes in 3 months, could also constitute recurrent diarrhea.

Chronic diarrhea : Here the onset of diarrhea is more insidious and usually less watery in nature. The stools are usually semisolid but larger in quantity and just about 4-5 times per day. As the disease is not dramatic in nature, the mother may find it very difficult to exactly date the onset of diarrheal symptoms. This type of syndrome is more often seen in children above 3 years of age although it may be seen at any age. Occasionally, the stools may be bulky and foul smelling but in large majority of children with chronic diarrhea, biochemical evidence of malabsorption may not be demonstrable. These children may also have intermittent episodes of frequent watery stools which may be confused with the syndrome of recurrent diarrhea.

While evaluating the history of a child with recurrent diarrhea, it is important to especially ask for the history of stools (type, frequency etc.) *in between* the episodes i.e. during the so-called "normal" period. In children with chronic diarrhea/malabsorption syndrome the stools are bulky, frequent (3-4 hrs), sticky and foul smelling, even during the so-called 'normal' periods. On the other hand, stools are completely normal in intervening period in children with recurrent diarrhea.

Malabsorption syndrome

Most text books of Pediatrics, describe chronic diarrhea under the heading of malabsorption syndrome (MAS) often using the two terms interchangeably. Malabsorption syndrome refers to a condition where there is biochemical evidence of malabsorption of one or more constituents of food. The typical malabsorption stools (bulky, oily, smelly) are produced when malabsorption of fats predominates. On the other hand, carbohydrate malabsorption may present as watery diarrhea.

It should be clearly understood that chronic diarrhea and malabsorption are not synonymous with each other. Each can exist without the other one. Most cases of chronic diarrhea do not have typical steatorrhic (large, bulk, foul smelling) stools. However, demonstration of type and extent of malabsorption existing in a child with diarrhea may help in delineating the exact cause of chronic diarrhea and/or malabsorption syndrome (Pancreatic or intestinal) and in planning rational therapy.

PERSISTENT DIARRHEA

Risk factors

The exact cause as to why an episode of diarrhea may get prolonged is not known. A variety of risk factors have been identified (Table 3.1) which seem to predispose the child to the possibility of developing persistent diarrhea. In a recent study, young age (< 6 months) and poor nutritional status of the host emerged as the ma-

Table 3.1. Risk factors in persistent diarrhea

Host factors	Young age (< 1 year) Malnutrition, Micronutrient (Zinc deficiency) Impaired cell mediated immunity Previous persistent diarrhea Recurrent acute diarrhea?
Preillness feeding practices	Non-breast fed, recent introduction of animal milk?
Stool pathogens	Enteroadherent or Enteroaggre-gative E. coli, EPEC Shigella
Drugs used in acute phase	Antibiotics

jor factors. Early curtailment of breast feeding and introduction of top milk were also very important factors apart from history of recurrent diarrhea in the past.

Etiopathogenesis : Hypothesis (Fig. 3.1)

Known risk factors and other known epidemiological characteristics regarding persistent diarrhea, can possibly be explained by an interaction of malnutrition and infection leading to intestinal mucosal damage which may lead to absorption of foreign (cow's milk) proteins and consequent hyper-sensitization.

Data from various studies including our own, suggest that occurrence of diarrhea in a malnourished young infant (< 6 months) who is already on top milk, is much more likely to get prolonged. Introduction of top milk (with contaminated bottles) introduces them to pathogenic bacteria and foreign proteins (cow's milk protein) at an age when the mucosa is still permeable to the proteins. Also, it predisposes them to occurrence of recurrent gut infection. Absorption of proteins may lead to the sensitization to these foreign proteins, which may be responsible for occurrence of post enteritis milk intolerance seen in many cases of persistent diarrhea. Whether

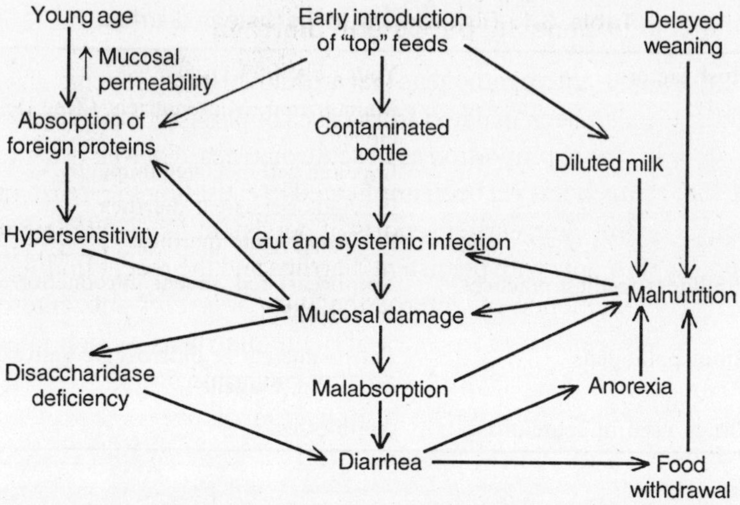

Fig. 3.1. Hypothesis to explain interplay of risk factors in persistent diarrhea.

due to infection (because of contaminated bottle) or because of hypersensitivity, this early weaned child gets recurrent diarrhea.

Malnutrition *per se* not only predisposes to increased incidence of diarrhea but also tends to prolong the course of disease. Various factors including decreased replenishment of damaged gut mucosa, may be responsible for increased duration of diarrhea in malnourished children.

Co-existing zinc deficiency, which is present in most of malnourished children may also play an important role in perpetuating the diarrhea.

Prevailing practices of diarrheal management viz. indiscriminate use of antibiotics and withholding of milk and other foods or giving of diluted milk, can lead to further compromise of nutritional status, and thus the vicious diarrhea-malnutrition-diarrhea cycle is set up, leading to ultimate development of persistent/protracted diarrhea and severe malnutrition.

Enteropathogens in persistent diarrhea

Almost all the enteropathogens that are known to cause acute diarrhea have also been isolated from cases of persistent diarrhea in roughly the same proportion as in acute diarrhea. Thus no definite enteropathogen has yet been implicated in causation of persistent diarrhea. However, earlier reports of persistent *Esch. coli* in gut mucosa of infants with persistent diarrhea and the recent findings of higher incidence of enteroadhesive *Esch. coli* and entero aggregative *Esch. coli* in cases of acute diarrheas, which later become prolonged, suggests that at least certain strains of *Esch. coli* may be responsible for the prolongation of diarrheal episodes in some children. Exact pathogenesis of diarrheal persistence due to these strains of *Esch. coli* is not known. They may be interferring with mucosal regeneration. Similarly in our experience and in experience of others, isolation of non-typhoidal *salmonella* in a case of acute diarrhea, is an alert signal for the development of persistent diarrhea in the infant.

Shigellosis has also been blamed for persistent diarrhea. However, it should be remembered that even after disappearance of blood from stool, after 2-3 days of antibiotics, it may take upto 3-4 weeks for stool frequency to return to normal in these children. During this apparent "persistence", child is usually active, non-anorexic and able to maintain hydration and nutrition if fed properly.

Rota virus is the commonest enteropathogen in acute diarrhea and could concievably be considered a cause of persistent diarrhea as it causes diarrhea by inflicting jejunal mucosal damage. However, a recent controlled study by us failed to demonstrate any role of Rota virus in causation of persistent diarrhea.

Systemic Infection in Persistent Diarrhea

Various studies have shown that 30-50% of children hospitalised with persistent diarrhea may have systemic infections at the time of admission. In fact, it is extremely difficult to exclude systemic infections in most of these cases as they are often moribund, and in our experience as many as 70-75% of these cases may end up receiving systemic antibiotics. Recently WHO protocol suggests that all children with severe malnutrition (body weight < 60%) and diarrhea should receive systemic antibiotics. The usual infections are U.T.I., pneumonias and septicemias. As most of the hospitalised children are severely malnourished, the systemic infections are often asymptomatic, and require careful screening for diagnosis.

Whether systemic infections by themselves predispose a diarrheal episode to become persistent or occurrence of systemic infection just precipitates admission in a child with persistent diarrhea, is more difficult to answer. However, our studies have clearly shown that presence of systemic infection at the time of onset of acute diarrhea, does not influence the duration of diarrhea i.e. they were not responsible for prolongation or protraction of diarrheal episodes. Nevertheless, a significant proportion of infants with protracted diarrhea at the time of hospitalization have systemic infections. Thus it appears that systemic infections are acquired later and only serve to precipitate hospitalisation of children with persistent diarrhea.

OTHER ETIOLOGICAL FACTORS

Apart from possible role of enteropathogens, a large number of specific conditions may be responsible for causation of persistent diarrhea but altogether they can be identified in a very small number of these cases and despite detailed studies, no etiological factor may be identified in as many as 40-70% cases.

Majority of persistent diarrheal episodes have six underlying factors (Table 3.2). It may be difficult to delineate a single factor in a given case as in majority of cases, multiple factors are operative, perhaps perpetuating each other. Studies at our centre have revealed that 3 or more of these factors are present in 40% of cases.

Table 3.2. Common underlying Pathogenic Factors Discernible in Cases of Persistent Diarrhea

Systemic infection
Malnutrition, PEM, Vitamin A, Zinc deficiency
Mucosal damage
Lactose intolerance
Colitis/antibiotic colitis
Cow's milk protein intolerance

Additionally the role of disturbed bile acid metabolism and altered gastrointestinal flora need to be kept in mind while planning the management of a child with protracted diarrhea. It will be appropriate to briefly discuss these underlying factors before discussing the management of protracted diarrhea.

Lactose intolerance : Lactose intolerance is the most common sugar intolerance seen in children with persistent diarrhea, although uncommonly sucrose or very rarely glucose intolerance can also occur. This is because lactase enzyme is present in the most superficial layers of jejunal mucosa and hence most vulnerable to damage. Lactose intolerance may be noticed in the first 2-3 days of a watery diarrhea episode more so in Rota virus cases but at this stage this is usually not of much importance as it tends to be mild and transitory, not even warranting milk withdrawl in majority of cases. On the other hand, lactose intolerance appearing after 5-7 days of diarrheal episode usually warrants more active management. Overall incidence is about 15-20% in *hospitalised protracted* diarrhea cases, being much more in malnourished children. It is uncommon among well nourished children with some prolongation of diarrhea - which is the condition most often seen in outpatient settings.

Suggestive clinical history (watery, explosive, frequent stools with red bottom) coupled with demonstration of reducing substances (++ or more) and reduced pH (< 5.5) in freshly passed stools (within

15-30 minutes), is usually sufficient to establish a diagnosis of lactose intolerance.

Lactose intolerance is a quantitative and not an "all or none" phenomenon. Occurrence of diarrhea depends upon the amounts of lactose ingested. Hence even reduction of dietary lactose (rather than complete elimination) often helps in overcoming the problem. Reduction in lactose content of an infant's diet can be achieved by mixing milk with cereals and reducing the total amounts of milk to about 30-50 ml/kg/day. This can also be achieved by giving curd (lactose content about 70% of milk) in diet, instead of milk. The food can be made energy dense by adding suitable amounts of vegetable oils to the diet.

Cow's milk protein intolerance (CMPI) : This is a rather controversial entity. There is a sharp divide between proponents and opponents of this condition, the later maintaining that the condition is extremely rare. The difficulty is further compounded by the fact that it is extremely difficult to establish the diagnosis of CMPI in clinical practice. 3 challenges criteria of Goldman, or 3 jejunal biopsy criteria of Iyangakaran et al. are both difficult to fulfil. Recently it has been suggested that demonstration of jejunal mucosal damage in a child with protracted diarrhea on milk, may be sufficient to diagnose cow's milk intolerance. This has been labelled as cow's milk elimination responsive enteropathy (CMERE) and can be demonstrated in upto 10-14% cases of protracted diarrhea. It is not clear whether these children represent true milk protein intolerance, but nevertheless these children do seem to require a temporary withdrawal (upto 4-6 weeks) of milk feeds from their diet. Even this requires at least one small intestine mucosal biopsy, a facility which is but rarely available in clinical practice. Demonstration of eosinophils in rectal biopsies (which can be obtained on an outpatient basis) has been suggested as an indirect evidence for CMPI and it may be a worthwhile exercise to get a rectal biopsy if the clinical suspicion is strong.

It may be difficult to distinguish C.M.P.I. from lactose intolerance as clinical features may overlap and both may exist together. Also the management used for one of them (like soya milk) may be useful for both of them.

Children who intolerant to cow's milk are also intolerant to buffalo's milk, though they may tolerate goat's milk quite well.

In clinical practice, cow's milk protein intolerance can be suspected when the diarrheal episode in a top fed child has exceeded more than 2-3 weeks, causing failure to thrive and if it does not respond to low lactose foods (curd, *khichri*). A trial of milk withdrawl and substitution of diet with other (non milk) protein sources (Rice- Dal-oil diet or soya milk) results in remission of diarrheal episodes but reintroduction of milk in diet causes recurrence of diarrhea, then it could be a case of CMPI. Although theoretically these children could also represent just lactose intolerance, yet the fact remains that it is nearly impossible to distinguish between the two conditions and quite often the two may coexist. A useful pointer to distinguish between the two is, that while in milk protein intolerance, the child gets diarrhea even on a small amounts of milk or milk products (curd, paneer etc.), in lactose intolerance, the child is often able to tolerate reduced amounts of milk in diet (e.g. curd, or milk with cereal mixtures). When faced with the clinical possibility of either lactose or CMP intolerance, it is practical to reduce milk content (thus reducing the total amounts of lactose) in diet and if the diarrhea is still not controlled, to think of CMPI and then completely withdraw milk and milk products.

In our clinical experience, CMPI is a very uncommon condition. In fact we have seen many children getting malnourished because of milk withdrawl due to alleged CMPI. In any case even infants with proven CMPI, tends to get better after 2 years of age.

Systemic infections : Although it may be difficult to pin point the role of systemic infections like pneumonia, U.T.I. etc. in causation of protracted diarrhea but it is clear that upto 30-50% of children with protracted diarrhea can be demonstrated to have systemic infections. Often these infections tend to be occult and children need to be carefully screened to detect and appropriately manage them. X-ray chest, Mantoux, urine culture, blood counts and blood cultures should be considered routine investigations in all such children and should be obtained prior to initiation of antibiotic therapy. As almost all hospitalised children with protracted diarrhea are severely malnourished and systemic infections are difficult to exclude, almost all these children may end up receiving antibiotics.

Persistent gut infection : Enteroadhesive and enteroaggregative *Esch. coli* have been held responsible for persistent diarrhea in some cases. However, It is not clear, whether these infections would require antibiotics or not and whether the required antibiotics would be systematically acting ones or locally acting ones. Controlled trials with oral gentamycin (15 mg/kg/day orally) or a combination of gentamycin and metronidazole, in cases of protracted diarrhea have not shown any consistent benefits.

We strongly believe that because these enteropathogens are highly adhering or attached to the gastrointestinal mucosa, they are like the weeds which grow on the bank of a river and as no amounts of "weedcides" put into the river will help to control the weeds growing on the banks, similarly antibiotics given orally are unlikely to have any affect on the entero-aggregative or entero-adhesive Eschericia Coli and they can probably be only managed with systemic antibiotics and with overall improvement in host resistance by improving his nutritional status; and by regeneration of mucosa.

In some Indian studies *Salmonella typhimurium* has been shown to be associated with persistent diarrhea. These children do not require antibiotics, unless the organism is present in blood.

Mucosal damage : Although not possible to obtain in non-hospitalised cases, jejunal or duodenal biopsy is helpful in diagnosis and management of these children. Presence and extent of mucosal damage seems to be an important prognostic factor in children with protracted diarrhea. Lebanthal considered mucosal damage as central (or "final common pathway") to the syndrome of persistent diarrhea.

Persistent mucosal damage or inadequate repair after an acute diarrheal episode, seems to be the single most important factor in persistence of a diarrheal episode. The mucosal damage itself may lead to multiple absorptive defects, persistence of diarrhea and worsening of nutritional status. Compromised nutritional status particularly zinc deficiency, itself may interfere with mucosal recovery. In various studies presence and severity of mucosal damage has emerged as the most important prognostic factor in cases of persistent diarrhea.

Mucosal damage itself may be due to persistent gut infection or due to an immune mediated injury. The later may be caused due to the development of hypersensitivity to ingested dietary proteins. As most of the patients of persistent diarrhea are young infants consuming mostly milk feeds, development of hypersensitivity to cow's (or buffalo's) milk protein is most commonly implicated in development of persistent diarrhea. Absorption of intact milk proteins through damaged mucosa leads to development of antibodies to milk protein which then perpetuate mucosal damage, setting up a type-II (b) immunological reaction.

Patchy enteropathy may suggest cow's milk protein intolerance while subtotal villous atrophy may even suggest celiac disease as the underlying cause.

Colitis : Almost 1/3rd of the cases described in the original series of Avery *et al.* had colitis or enterocolitis. Even in our series of 76 cases, evidence of colitis was present in almost 20% cases as suggested by presence of red cells and/or pus cells (> 20/H.P.F.) in stool, and with histopathological evidence of colitis. In most cases it is infective in origin, although uncommonly antibiotic induced colitis can also be seen. Infective colitis in a severely malnourished child or in infants less than 6 months of age would usually require systemic antibiotics.

Antibiotic colitis : Occasionally broad spectrum antibiotics used (mostly unwarranted) for diarrhea (or other illnesses) can themselves lead to occurrence of a colitis. Ampicillin, Chloramphenicol, Cephalosporins are the usual offending drugs, although almost any antibiotic or chemotherapeutic agent may be responsible. The cause of this type of colitis has been traced to the overgrowth of an anaerobic bacteria, *Clostridium difficile* and liberation of an enterotoxin by this organism. The diagnosis can be established by either demonstrating toxin in the serum or stool or by growing *Clostridium* in the stool. As both of these facilities are rarely available even at referral hospitals, the entity has to be considered and diagnosed on clinical grounds. It is important to do so, as continuation (or addition of other antibiotics) may further worsen the colitis and even prove fatal.

The diagnosis of antibiotic colitis can be suspected on clinical grounds when the child's diarrhea, *after initial improvement*, increases or becomes invasive (pus cells/red cells in stools) after 4-5 days use of antibiotics. Initially atleast, the child looks otherwise well, taking his feeds. But soon, if appropriate action is not taken, the child becomes moribund, refusing to feed and developing abdominal distension and passage of blood and pus in stools. If available, sigmoidoscopy may be done and a rectal biopsy obtained. Diagnosis depends on a high index of suspicion and should be strongly considered in all infants who develop or worsen their diarrhea on antibiotics, after initial improvement.

However, despite widespread use of antibiotics in our country, we have been able to establish the diagnosis of antibiotic colitis in very few children. In fact most of the so-called hospital acquired (children already on antibiotics) diarrhea with pus cells and red cells in stools, turn out to have *Salmonella typhimurium* infections rather than antibiotic colitis. These children mostly require stoppage of antibiotics. Also we have seen more cases of resistant (persistant) Shigella dysentery rather than that of antibiotic colitis.

Poor nutritional status : Malnutrition in the host is also an important underlying factor in causing persistent diarrhea. Most studies show that the average duration of an acute diarrheal episode is longer in a malnourished child compared to that in a normal nourished child. Increased gut contamination due to proliferation of non specific bacteria and decreased mucosal enzymes due to persistent mucosal damage may be important factors causing prolongation of diarrheal disease in malnourished state. In fact, the poor nutritional status, and the need to restore the nutritional status, in these children, has recently been recognised to be of such crucial importance in infants with protracted diarrhea, that many workers refer to diarrhea as a "nutritional disease". Not only malnutrition prolongs the duration of diarrhea, but diarrheal illness itself helps to worsen the nutritional status, thus setting up the vicious malnutrition diarrhea-malnutrition cycle (Fig. 2.1, pp 28).

These children often have multiple vitamin and mineral deficiencies apart from protein-energy malnutrition.

Zinc deficiency is particularly prevalent in children with protracted diarrhea and needs to be tackled vigorously. In fact zinc deficiency is believed to be a major causative factor in prolongation of diarrheal episode. Addition of zinc in therapeutic regimes has helped in curtailing the duration and improving the outcome of diarrhea.

MANAGEMENT

Epidemiologically, around 10% of all acute diarrheal episodes tend to persist beyond 14 days. However, majority of these episodes represent only a normal variation in natural history of different etiological agents. A study has shown that 10% of even Rotavirus diarrhea may last for as long as 21 days but may have no other clinical problems. The frequency and consistency of stools following *shigella* infection very often lasts for several days following acute illness. Hence mere prolongation of diarrhea episode should not become a cause of worry. Attempt should be made to delineate those episodes which are associated with weight loss as these are the very cases which are likely to have a bad outcome. Studies have shown that only 10% of all prolonged diarrheal episodes may have associated weight loss (become protracted).

Persistent diarrheal episodes, especially those associated with failure to thrive, present a major therapeutic challenge to pediatricians today. The greatest difficulty in managing these children arises from the fact, that unlike other conditions, in most cases of persistent diarrhea a single etiological factor cannot be held responsible for the particular episode. In fact in majority of the episodes, multiple factors are operative as pointed above. Furthermore, most of these children are quite moribund requiring urgent therapeutic intervention, even while the diagnostic work-up is underway.

Diarrhea of 7-14 days duration

Average duration of acute diarrhea is 3-5 days and most diarrheal episodes resolve within 7 days. Parents get unduly worried when the diarrhea persists even beyond 3 to 5 days. They pester the physician for action and many of us succumb to these pressures. As stated above, even in natural history of acute diarrhea many episodes of diarrhea may last beyond 7 days normally, and hence do not require management on the lines of persistent diarrhea. In general approach to a child with diarrhea of 7-14 days duration is similar to that to children of > 14 days duration, remembering that majority of these episodes only represent natural prolongation of diarrhea and episode without any complication.

It is important to maintain nutritional and hydration status during this period and to avoid drugs (unless absolutely warranted) and dietary manipulations during this stage. Some children may have clinical and laboratory evidence of lactose intolerance even at such an early stage of diarrheal disease, but as pointed above, this usually warrants no energetic management.

Unless alert signals are present (Table 3.3), these children can be easily managed at home. Foods like curd, banana, mashed potatoes, *Khichri, Dalia* etc. should be given in large amounts to meet the increased calorie demands during this time together with continued breast feeding. Low lactose foods like milk based cereal diets (*Suji ki kheer, Dudh ka Dalia* etc.) can help to decrease the lactose load while continuing to provide adequate calories. Addition of edible oils in the cereal diet can greatly increase the calorie density of food and help in maintaining nutritional balance. Top milk may be required to be restricted (30-50 ml/kg/day) but should not be replaced by Soyamilk. Remember the incidence of soya protein intolerance following acute diarrhea, is almost 15 times more than that of cow's milk protein intolerance and hence in no case should soya milk be introduced in the diet of a child with diarrheal episode of less than 14 days duration.

Table 3.3. Alert signals warranting hospitalisation in children with diarrhea 7-14 days duration

Severe malnutrition
Weight loss occurring during diarrheal episode
Unable to maintain hydration/nutrition
Persistent anorexia
Systemic infection (persistent pyrexia localising signs)

Antibiotics (local or systemic) also do not seem to have much role in this situation unless evidence of frank colitis or a systemic infection is present. If the evidence of colitis is present after a few days of the onset of diarrheal episode and the child is already on antibiotics, then it may be a case of antibiotic associated colitis and hence in these children, withdrawal of antibiotics and if required administration of oral metronidazole (20 mg/kg) or Vancomycin may be helpful.

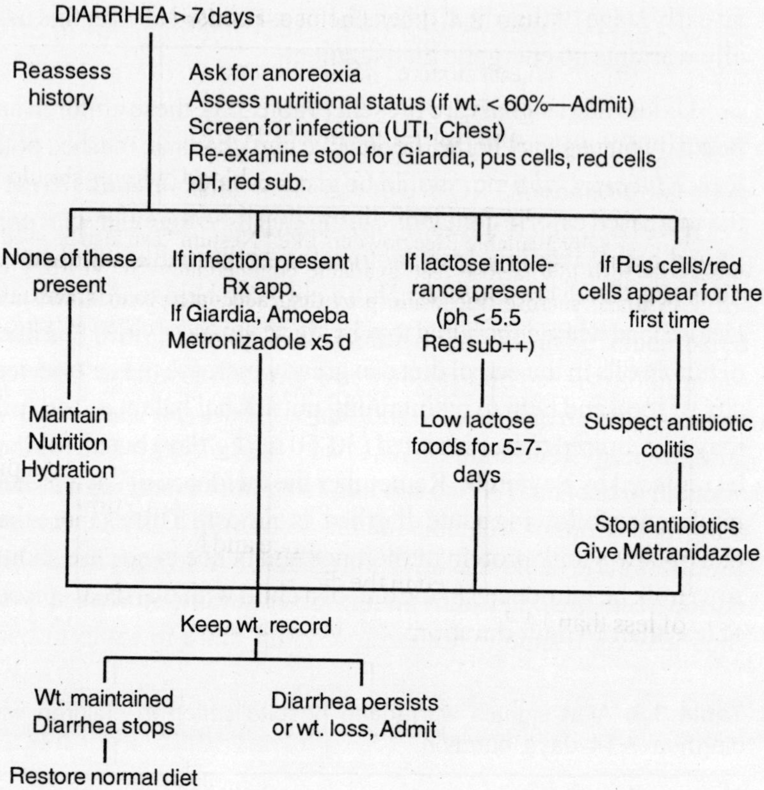

Fig. 3.2. Clinical approach to a child with diarrhea of 7-14 days duration.

It is important to monitor weight daily, to be sure that the child is maintaining adequate weight gain, despite continued diarrhea. This will also help greatly in reassuring the parents.

Diarrhea beyond 14 days or that associated with weight loss

Children with diarrhea of > 14 days and no alert signals (Table 3.3) can also be managed on the same lines as mentioned above.

However, when a child presents with a prolonged diarrheal

Table 3.4. Low Lactose Foods

Milk cereal (Rice*, Wheat) mixture
Curd
Curd/Cereal mixture (Rice*, Wheat etc.)
Meshed Bananas

N.B. Commercially available Rice powders like "Nestum" can also be used. Lactodex is also low lactose feed available commercially. Simyl MCT is also lactose and sucrose free while providing adequate proteins and fats in the form of medium chain triglycerides which are better observed across a damaged mucosa.

* For infants 5 gms of boiled rice may be added to 75 ml of milk and made up to 100 ml. With added sugar it will give a calorie density of 0.7 Cal/ml and will still be liquid in consistency.

** For older infants and children, the amount of Rice can be increased to 10 gms to increase the calorie density to 1 Cal/ml with a semisolid consistency. Curd can also be used in place of milk.

episode with weight loss, he should be hospitalised. It is important to do so, as these children can have an unpredictable course and may become serious at any time. Further they would require repeated investigations which may not be feasible in an out-patient situation.

After admission it is necessary to take a detailed history regarding the onset, duration, character of stools at the onset and any subsequent change, associated features like anorexia, fever, cough, urine, frequency etc. and the management received (drugs, diet etc.) till then. Physical examination of the child should include assessment of nutritional and hydration status and careful screening for any associated infections (CSOM, pneumonia and even meningitis).

These children should be viewed more as severely malnourished infants with prolonged diarrhea, rather than as cases of persistent diarrhea with malnutrition. This approach will help to focus diagnostic approach and management to the child as a whole rather than only frequent passage of stools.

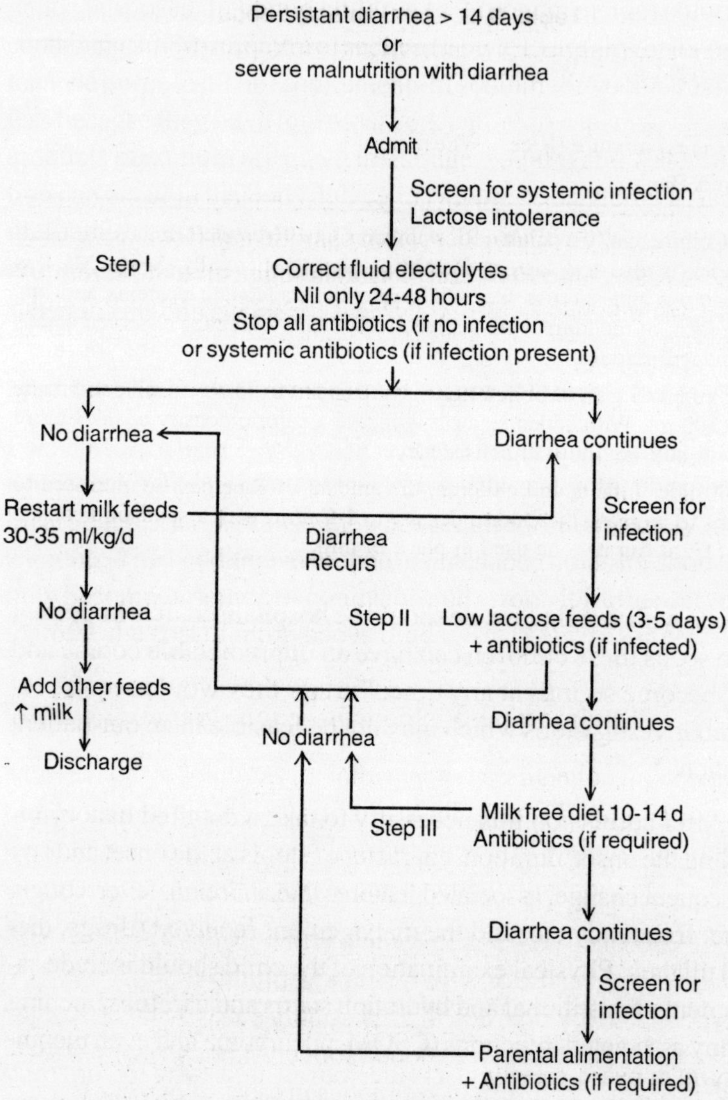

Fig. 3.3. Algorithm for management of persistent diarrhea.

Preliminary investigations should include stool examination for pus cells, ova, cysts and red cells and for pH and reducing substances. A total and differential leucocyte counts including band cells counts and blood culture should also be obtained. A urine examination and culture (if required) and an X-ray chest should be obtained in all cases. Stool cultures have no value as organisms grown in routine culture of stool may not necessarily be enteropathogens and hence their antibiotic sensitivity also has no implication in choosing antibiotics. If available, stool osmolarity and electrolytes may be obtained. A stool osmotic gap (total osmolarity-2 x Sodium content) of less than 50 is suggestive of secretory diarrhea, which may require treatment for sepsis and prolonged parenteral nutrition. This may also be a signal for searching for rare causes like VIPoma, ganglion-neuronoma or congenital microvillous atrophy.

In large majority of cases of protracted diarrhea, no single etiological diagnosis is possible. These children are often moribund with fluid, electrolyte and nutritional imbalance and their management must be started immediately while the results of investigations are being awaited. A stepwise approach is discussed below :

Step I : If the clinical examination and preliminary investigations fail to reveal any evidence of systemic infection, then it would be prudent to stop all antibiotics and stop oral feeds for 24-48 hrs and maintain hydration with intravenous fluids. Usually the diarrhea would tend to subside with these measures alone and the oral feeding can be restarted beginning with oral rehydration solution and later with gradual regrading (initially small amounts of undiluted milk and then gradually full amounts of milk). However, if the diarrhea does not settle down even on I.V. fluids and nil orally, it suggests a secretory diarrhea. This is usually due to persistent gut infection or rare causes as mentioned above. Although no consensus exists regarding the use of antibiotics in cases of persistent gut infection, but a trial may be warranted with systemic antibiotics in these cases, especially as most of the cases are as such malnourished and have a high incidence of systemic infections.

Step II : If the diarrhea recurs on reintroduction of milk feeds, one should suspect secondary lactose intolerance besides possibility of systemic infection. The child may need to be rescreened for systemic infection and treated appropriately. Even if no biochemical evidence of lactose intolerance is present, it is advisable to give low lactose diet to these children and continue the same for at least 5-7 days (unless the diarrhea worsens). If the child tolerates low lactose diet and starts gaining weight on the same, the amount of milk and other foods can be slowly increased in diet.

Step III: However, if the child fails to tolerate even low lactose feeds (about 20-25% of hospitalised protracted diarrhea children would do so) then the clinical setting suggests possibility of CMPI besides possibility of a systemic infection. Thus when low lactose diet also fails, it is best to omit milk and milk products completely from diet and instead to give complete milk free diets (Table 3.5) like Soyamilk, Rice-Dal-oil (Table 3.6) diet or amylase rich Rice dal diet (Table 3.7), besides treating systemic infection if present. This is successful in most of these cases, thus leaving only 1-2% cases of protracted diarrhea, who fail to respond to these measures. If available special milks like Nutramigen or Prosobee can be used as milk free diet - but these are extremely costly.

Table 3.5. Lactose and milk protein free diet

- Soya milk (Nusobee, Soyal, Prosoyal, Isomil)
- Rice-Dal-Oil Diet
- Amylase rich rice dal diet
- Nutramigen
- Pregestemil
- Comminuted chicken

Table 3.6 : Rice Dal Oil Diet

- Rice 50 gms
- Dal 30 gms
- Salt 1 tsf. in 1 litre of water
- Sugar 4 tsf. and then add 30 gms of oil (preferably coconut oil)

Table 3.7. Amylase rich rice dal diet

A. Preparing Amylase Powder

Wheat grains (Handful)
↓
Soak and keep in wet muslin cloth for 48 hrs.
↓
Germinating wheat
↓
Take out the shoot
↓
Sun dry (8 hrs.) or oven dry 4 hrs.
↓
Grind and make fine powder (amylase rich flour)
↓
Store in air tight container (for upto 1 month)
(Avoid humidity)

B. Preparing Amylase Rich Rice Dal Diet

20 gm Rice, 5 gm Dal, 100 ml water
↓ Cook
Thick Paste
↓ Cool to room temperature
Add 1 tsf of amylase powder and a pinch of salt
↓
Wait for 15-20 minutes
↓
Liquifies - ready for feeding as Amylase rich diet (1 Kcal/ml)

Once the child responds to completely milk free diet, then it is advisable to persist with the same diet for at least 4-6 weeks. Also milk should be reintroduced in their diets in a very careful manner and under supervised conditions. Occasionally these infants may require milk free diet for as long as 8-12 months.

Vitamin and mineral supplementation especially zinc should be given to ensure normal intake.

Step IV : If the child is unable to tolerate even Rice dal or amylase rich diet or soya milk and continues to have diarrhea, then the child would require parenteral alimentation. Now-a-days both intravenous lipid and aminoacid preparations have become available in Indian market and hence can be used more frequently. Parenteral alimentation requires careful asepsis and calculations of proteins, calories, fluid and electrolyte requirements with clinical and biochemical monitoring. Carelessly carried out parenteral alimentation can prove more disasterous.

Thus overall efforts in a child with protracted diarrhea should be directed towards detecting and treating associated systemic infections and towards restoring nutritional status preferably by oral route and if required even by intravenous route. Systemic infections should be carefully looked for at each of the management step and treated appropriately. Food intolerance (like lactose and milk protein), if present, needs to be circumvented by appropriate dietary manipulations in a stepwise manner, to ensure proper nutritional intake. It is important to look at the child as a whole rather than the number of stools passed by him. Thus his appetite, nutritional intake and weight gain are more important factors to note rather than the number of stools. It is usually seen that the diarrhea controls itself as the nutritional status improves. In our experience treatment of systemic infections has greatly reduced the problems of dietary management of children with protracted diarrhea and improved the outcome remarkably (almost nil mortality).

Drugs in protracted diarrhea

Antibiotics : As systemic and/or persistent gut infections (as suggested by secretory diarrhea) are fairly common in children with protracted diarrhea and often these malnourished children are moribund on admission where septicemia cannot be excluded, many of these children require appropriate antibiotic therapy. In our experience almost 70-80% hospitalized cases of persistent diarrhea require systemic antibiotics, although systemic infection can be demonstrated only in 30-35% of cases. As per WHO protocol, all severely malnourished children with diarrhea (irrespective of duration) would require systemic antibiotics. As most children with persistent diarrhea are severely malnourished, it is easy to see why most of these children end up receiving antibiotics.

The choice of antibiotic is determined by the site of infection and probable etiological agent, remembering again that the organisms (or their sensitivity) cultured from stool have no significance in management. A combination of first (Cefazolin) or third (Cefotaxime/Ceftriaxone) generation cephalosporin together with an aminoglycoside (gentamycin/amikacin) offers a good choice esp. when septicemia is suspected. Occasionally response to even these antibiotics may be inadequate and then drugs like ciprofloxacin or ofloxacin may be required. Oral antibiotics have not been shown to be of any use in these cases.

Zinc : Oral zinc supplementation 10-20 mg/day, has been shown to definitely decrease the duration of diarrhea in these children. This must be given to all such cases for 14 days..

Lopremide : Antimotility and antisecretory drugs like lopremide, have been used by some in protracted diarrhea without much success. As such, its harmful side effects far outweigh its possible usefulness. Even if used, its dose should not exceed 0.4 mg/kg/day and that too for a short period of time. Currently its use in children is banned and liquid preparations are no longer available.

Cholestyramine : Altered intestinal bile salt composition may be responsible for malabsorption and persistence of diarrhea in a few cases. Cholestyramine has been used in selected cases of protracted diarrhea with limited benefits. Large doses (4 to 6 gm, daily) are required, irrespective of age, and still the benefits are only marginal and debatable.

Lactobacilli or Probiotics : Indiscriminate use of antibiotics may lead to alteration of gut flora with emergence of predominantly resistant bacteria. *Lactobacilli* preparations may help by re-establishing non-pathogenic lactobacilli in the gut and in overcoming the pathogenic bacteria. However, avoidance of antibiotics and encouragement of breast feeding will greatly avoid the necessity of using artificial *lactobacilli* preparations of doubtful use. Despite claims to the contrary, the effectiveness of *lactobacilli* is compromised with simultaneous use of oral broad spectrum antibiotics and hence this should be avoided (see also chapter on drugs in diarrhea).

Metronidazole : Prolonged diarrhea in adults is often due to amebiasis and hence antiamebic drugs are frequently used in general practice. Therefore, practitioners are also often tempted to use these drugs, (either alone or in combination with antibiotic or chemotherapeutic agents) in infants also. However, none of studies in infant's protracted diarrhea have demonstrated amebiasis or giardiasis as significant pathogens. Hence metronidazole or other similar drugs (entamizole etc.) have no role in protracted diarrhea as such, unless warranted by demonstration of giardial/amoebic trophozoites in stool.

Occasionally, however, the protracted diarrhea could occur because of *antibiotic associated colitis*. Increase or recurrence of diarrhea with or without evidence of pus cell, red cell etc. in stool, after 4-5 days of antibiotics in acute diarrhea, suggests antibiotic colitis on clinical grounds. In these children, withdrawl of offending antibiotics is usually sufficient to control the diarrhea. Occasionally these children may also require metronidazole (20 mg/kg/day for 5 days) or vancomycin for taking care of the anaerobic bacteria, *Clostridrium deficile*, which has been established as the cause of antibiotic colitis.

Thus, it would be seen that majority of drugs (except systemic antibiotics and oral zinc supplementation) offer no advantage in cases of protracted diarrhea and the mainstay of its management is nutritional rehabilitation with commonly available household foods.

Proper nutritional support during acute diarrhea would hopefully prevent significant proportions of protracted diarrheal episodes.

RECURRENT DIARRHEA

Children with frequent diarrheal episodes can often masquerade clinically as cases of diarrhea of long duration. Only careful history helps to delineate that there are several distinct episodes separated by intervening normal periods rather than a single prolonged episode. In such cases, history of each episode should be taken carefully. Occasionally they would be found to be of different nature. This is not surprising as each of these episodes represent an occurrence of an acute diarrheal episode which may be due to different enteropathogens at different times. It is also quite possible that while initial episodes are of short duration, as frequency of episodes increase, their duration may also increase. Some of these children may later on present as chronic diarrhea.

Predisposing factors : Poor environmental sanitation, pre-disposes to repeated episodes of enteric infection. Early curtailment of breast feeding and introduction of bottle feeding, which are often contaminated or even early introduction of plain water (often itself contaminated) are also important micro-environmental factors predisposing to recurrent diarrhea. It is not surprising that majority of these episodes occur among preschool children of poor, illiterate families living in deprived, urban slums with abysmal levels of environmental sanitation.

Etiological agents : Almost all the etiological agents responsible for acute-diarrheal episodes can be responsible for different episodes of recurrent diarrhea in the same child.

Management

Each episodes of diarrhea should be approached and managed on similar lines as outlined for acute diarrhea earlier. Emphasis should be on maintaining hydration and nutrition. Extra nutritional supplements should be made available during convalescent period.

Nutritional status must be assessed carefully (measuring body weight on each visit and by plotting on a growth chart) and appropriate advice given for improving nutritional status, Vitamin and mineral supplementation, particularly iron and zinc (1-2 mg/kg/d) should also be given. If there is a persistent growth faltering (failure to gain weight) one should try to assess for underlying malabsorptive states like celiac disease (*vide infra*).

Advice also need to be given on ensuring dietary hygiene. As macroenvironmental issues like safe water supply, sanitary excreta disposal etc., are usually beyond the means of individual family, advice should concentrate on ensuring microenvironmental sanitation (Table 3.8). This includes advice on exclusive breast feeding (till at least 4 months of age), avoidance of bottles and giving of top milk by spoon, hand washing (by mother/child), storage of water under hygiene conditions at home and if possible, boiling of water for infant feeds and avoiding cold or stale weaning food (as they often get contaminated) for infant feeding.

Table 3.8. Microenvironmental measures helpful in decreasing incidence of recurrent diarrhea

Exclusive breast feeding till 4 month of age
Avoid bottle, give spoon feeds
Hand washing by mother/child
Store drinking water hygienically
Boil water or use filters
Give only freshly/adequately warmed foods - avoid stale/cold foods

Toddler's diarrhea : Irritable colon syndrome

Occasionally children suffering from Toddler's diarrhea (or irritable colon syndrome) may present clinically as recurrent diarrhea episodes. Each episodes is of variable severity and duration, almost never dehydrating the child and despite the long history of diarrhea these children (6 months to 2 years of age) are never malnourished and continue to gain weight adequately. Typically the consistency of stool varies greatly, being comparatively well formed in the morning becoming progressively watery by evening. There may be a history of acute diarrheal episode at the onset of illness.

Management of Toddler's diarrhea

These children are usually well nourished, belonging to comparatively better socio-economic status. These children tend to get worse on liquid diet and as milk is the major diet given at this age, it is not surprising that many of these children may be diagnosed as intolerant to milk. Obviously this diagnosis should not be applied loosely. It should be remembered that children with milk intolerance (CMPI) would tend to loose weight, while children with Toddler's diarrhea continue to gain weight adequately. Also children with CMPI will not tolerate even small amounts of milk, while children with Toddler's diarrhea may continue to do well on curd, paneer etc.

Management largely consists of parental assurance, decrease in liquid diet and increase in solid/semisolid foods in diet. Isabgol with curd also help to make the stool firmer. Most of these children would improve by 2 years of age. It is important not to unnecessarily withdraw milk (or other food items) from the diet as otherwise that itself may lead to nutritional deprivation.

CHRONIC DIARRHEA

Chronic diarrhea in older children usually has an insidious onset. The stools are semisolid and large, with only marginally increased frequency. Occasionally they may be bulky, fatty and foul smelling, suggesting fat malabsorption.

Even children with chronic diarrhea, may have intermittent history of apparently watery diarrhea mimicking recurrent diarrhea, but a carefully taken history would reveal that while the stools in intervening period are entirely normal (1-2 formed stools) in children with recurrent diarrhea, those continue to be abnormal (large, bulky, semisolid) in children with chronic diarrhea.

Further, chronic diarrhea and malabsorption syndrome are not synonymous. Most children with chronic diarrhea do not have typical bulky, greesy, sticky stools of fat malabsorption.

Etiological considerations

Although theoretically, a large number of conditions can give rise to chronic diarrhea with or without malabsorption, but the common causes seen in our practice are listed in Table 3.9

Table 3.9. Common causes of chronic diarrhea at L.N. Hospital, Delhi

Non-dysentric	*Dysentric*
Celiac disease	Amebic colitis
Tropical enteropathy	Ulcerative colitis
Giardiasis	Non-specific colitis
Intestinal tuberculosis	Tubercular colitis
AIDS	Crohn's disease
Irritable Bowel syndrome	
Short bowel syndrome	

As cystic fibrosis is not common in our country, chronic diarrhea due to pancreatic insufficiency is not common in our experience. In fact, in most cases of chronic diarrhea, biochemical evidence of fat malabsorption is not demonstrable.

Uncommon causes of chronic diarrhea include protein loosing enteropathy, abetalipoproteinemia, intestinal lymphangiectasis, autoimmune enteropathy etc. Worm infestation, often mentioned as cause of chronic diarrhea seems more coincidental than causal.

Clinical features

Clinical features of different entities are often overlapping. Nevertheless it is often possible to distinguish between different conditions by careful consideration of clinical features and by simple investigations.

Giardiasis

This can occur at any age. The stools are uncharacteristic but may be often bulky with peculiar smell. Uncommonly a "gastrocolic" pattern with formed stools (unlike Toddler's diarrhea gastrocolic pattern with watery stools) could be seen. Diagnosis can be achieved by doing repeated stool examination. Although the exact pathogenetic role of mere giardial cysts is not certain, yet if a symptomatic child is passing cysts in stools, it is prudent to treat with a course of metronidazole (20 mg/kg/d for 5 days). Occasionally a repeat course after a gap of 7-10 days may be required. Of course, if trophozoites are present, treatment must be given. Repeating stool examination in a cyst passer should be avoided, as it is likely that cysts may persist in stool although the diarrhea has recovered.

Tropical Enteropathy

Stool pattern may vary from recurrent watery diarrhea (each episode partially or completely responding to chemotherapeutic agents) to large, semiformed stools. Failure to thrive and even frank malnutrition is common. Usually preschool children are affected. D-xylose test is often abnormal and uncommonly, even fat malabsorption may also be present. Some authors have labelled this condition as "contaminated bowel syndrome". Severe forms may manifest as tropical sprue with frank evidence of malabsorption.

Diagnosis should be suspected clinically in a pre-school child, with frequent diarrheal episodes responding to some treatment (usually antibiotics) briefly and sooner or later relapsing and even producing malnutrition. Iron deficiency and/or folate deficiency anemia is common. If obtained, jejunal biopsy shows mild to moderate villous atrophy. In our experience this is a fairly common cause of chronic diarrhea esp. in preschool children coming *from deprived environmental circumstances*.

The management consists of nutritional supplementation including adequate calories and proteins, appropriate for age and nutritional status and advice on dietary hygiene. Folic acid supplementation (2.5 mg-5 mg/d) may be helpful as also zinc (2-3 mg/kg/d). A 6-12 weeks course of antibiotics (usually cotrimoxazole and metronidazole) helps greatly in these children. We have seen dramatic improvement in appetite, weight and stool pattern with this antibiotic regimen in these children, with reversal of mucosal damage. Clinical response to antibiotic treatment is seen within 15 days and if no response is obtained within 15 days, antibiotics should be stopped and alternative diagnosis should be looked for.

Tuberculosis

Intestinal tuberculosis can often present as chronic diarrhea in children. The text book description of alternating constipation and diarrhea is rarely seen in children and most common presentation of intestinal tuberculosis in children is with chronic diarrhea with or without abdominal pain. The clinical picture is indistinguishable from other causes and help has to be obtained from other evidences of tuberculosis (Mantoux, Chest X-ray, USG abdomen/Ba meal follow through and even CT scan) in the child. Thus all children with chronic diarrhea or recurrent abdominal pain should be carefully screened for tuberculosis.

Celiac disease

Chronic diarrhea due to gluten induced euteropathy is probably the commonest cause of chronic diarrhea in children seen at tertiary care centres with pediatric gastroenterology set up. Recent community based surveys from Delhi, Ludhiana etc. have revealed that the gluten hypersensitivity in Northern India may be as frequent as in Western Europe, USA etc. Thus, one out of every 200 to 400 children may have gluten hypersensitivity as shown by positive serological tests. Only a small number of these, generally predisposed individuals, actually develop clinical manifestations of celiac disease (celiac Iceberg).

Clinical manifestations

Clinical manifestation always begin after the introduction of wheat (biscuit, dalia, cerelac, roti, bread, etc.) in the diet. But there is variable period of time between the age at which the wheat is introduced in diet to the age at which symptoms may became manifest (time of onset). Usually symptoms start 3-4 months after the introduction of wheat in diet but may be delayed by as much as 3-4 years when the introduction of wheel in diet is delayed beyond infancy. Duration of breast feeding also influences the age of onset of symptoms. Longer the duration, later the manifestations. It is now believed that introduction of wheat, when the baby is still breast-fed, may help to prevent clinical manifestation of the disease.

Diarrhea usually begins insidiously and usually consists of 3-4 semi-loose stools per day. These semi-loose stools may be punctuated with episodes of watery diarrhea. It is uncommon to see typical steatorrhic stool i.e. large, bulky, green, foul smelling, sticky stools.

Apart from diarrhea, failure to thrive and anemia are other prominent features of celiac disease. Anemia typically responds poorly to iron supplementation or recurs soon after stoppage of iron supplementation.

Atypical manifestation

Children with celiac disease, may never manifest chronic diarrhea and may only present with anemia, failure to thrive, rickets, abdominal distension or short stature. Other atypical presentation includes delayed puberty.

Diagnosis

High index of suspicion is required. Any child with failure to thrive with or without diarrhea should be investigated for possibility of celiac disease. Serological tests like antitissue transglutaminase (anti TTGA) or anti-Endomysial antibodies (anti-EMA) are good screening tests with more than 90% sensitivity and 95% specificity.

However despite availability of highly specific serological tests, it must be remembered that the gold standard for diagnosis of celiac disease remains the histological demonstration of intestinal villous atrophy, by obtaining either endoscopic duodenal biopsy or jejunal biopsy.

Biochemical tests of malabsorption (D-Xylose, fat estimation in stool etc.) are useful but rarely available in clinical practice in a dependable manner and in any case, they only demonstrate inability of the intestine to absorb the particular nutrient without delineating the underlying cause.

Other Food Allergies

Although Western Text Books of Pediatrics mention allergy to many other foods (esp. milk) as a cause of chronic diarrhea, however, these are not commonly seen in tropical countries. Probably most problems in these countries arise because of food deprivation rather than due to food allergies! In any case, milk protein intolerance, if it occurs, tends to present more as a persistent/protracted diarrhea in infancy rather than as chronic diarrhea in older children.

Other causes of chronic diarrhea

Worms, esp. round worms, are often mentioned as causes of chronic diarrhea in tropical children. However, more recent studies have shown that worm infestations are no more frequent among diarrheal children than in non diarrheal children. Hence mere presence of *ascaris* ova in the stool of a child with chronic diarrhea should not make a clinician jump to a conclusion that chronic diarrhea is due to round worms. Occasionally *Trichuris trichura* may be responsible for chronic diarrhea, but this worm is rarely reported in Indian stools.

Cryptosporidium

This parasite is also mentioned as a cause of chronic diarrhea. It is predominantly a pathogen in immunocompromised host. The diarrhea can be quite severe and watery. In any case this is not a common pathogen in immunocompetent children with chronic diarrhea.

Acquired Immuno Deficiency Syndrome (AIDS)

This syndrome occurs due to HIV infection. This infection is assuming increasing frequency at least in certain parts of our country (Tamil Nadu, Maharashtra, Coastal Andhra Pradesh, North East States etc.). In children this is usually acquired perinatally from an infected mother. Clinical manifestations (including chronic diarrhea) usually start in late pre-school age or early-school age. Generalised lymphadeno-pathy, chronic diarrhea, weight loss, recurrent infections including tuberculosis are hallmarks of this disease. *Thus all children with chronic diarrhea and failure to thrive should be screened for HIV infection*. These children may also demonstrate intestinal mucosal atrophy (AIDS enteropathy) on biopsy. Today many anti-retroviral drugs are available for control of HIV infections and AIDS. Discussion of their use is beyond the scope of this book.

Cystic fibrosis

This is mentioned as a frequent cause of chronic diarrhea and malabsorption type of stools in Western text books, where this is a frequent problem. Although some cases of cystic fibrosis with pulmonary manifestations have been described in Indian children also, yet this does not appear to be an important cause of chronic diarrhea in our set up. If chronic diarrhea occurs, stools are more likely to be frankly steatorrehic (large, sticky, foul smelling) as in these children diarrhea is mostly because of pancreatic enzyme deficiency. Diagnosis can be confirmed by investigating sweat chloride of children. Management requires dietary supplementation with pancreatic enzymes (amylase, diastase) in large quantities.

Non-specific diarrhea

After excluding above mentioned causes of chronic diarrhea, one is left with about 15-20% children in whom no specific cause can be labelled in our set up. The stool pattern is varied in these children and nutritionally these children may remain largely unaffected. As the cause is not clear, so the treatment is only symptomatic. Dietary hygiene, adequate nutrition and correction of micronutrient (zinc, folate, iron, Vitamin-A) deficiency if any, is all that can usually be offered to manage these children. These children may require reinvestigations/referral to a specialist, if they continue to loose weight or have inadequate weight gain despite adequate nutritional intake.

Clinical Approach

When a child presents with chronic diarrhea, detailed history of the age of onset, type and content of stools, any associated problems and history of weaning etc. should be carefully obtained. On physical examination, any evidence of failure to thrive (decreased weight for age) and nutritional deficiencies should be carefully recorded. As occasionally liver disease can also present as chronic diarrhea, the size and consistency of liver should also be carefully recorded.

Routine investigations should include (i) repeated stool examination for ova and cyst, (ii) Mantoux test, (iii) complete hemogram including E.S.R. (ix) X-ray chest and (v) routine urine examination and if required urine culture and sensitivity.

If available D-xylose test for malabsorption should be obtained as also 72 hour fecal fat. Evidence of fat malabsorption can be seen by looking for fat droplets on microscopic examination of stools, which look like air vacuoles on routine examination. They can be stained with Sudan III dye when they are seen as orange colour droplets. Presence of more than 3-5 such droplets per high power field correlates well with biochemical evidence of fat malabsorption.

If celiac disease is suspected, screening serological tests (antigliadin, antiendomysial, anti-tissue transglutaminase antibodies) should be obtained.

If any of the investigations is abnormal, action need to be taken on the lines suggested by the abnormal investigations. It may be very difficult to establish the diagnosis of intestinal tuberculosis but all efforts must be made to make this diagnosis. USG abdomen, Barium meal follow through and occasionally, even CT scan can be required for this purpose, not forgetting the usefulness of Mantoux test and X-ray chest in these children.

If all those investigations are normal and there is no failure to thrive, then parents should be reassured and given advise for diet and hygiene. Close follow-up should be maintained to ensure that the child is gaining weight adequately.

Even when the investigations are normal, but the child is having failure to thrive (weight loss or inadequate weight gain), then it is prudent to refer the child to a pediatric gastroenterology unit for a jejunal/endoscopic duodenal biopsy. However, if these facilities do not exist, in view of the fact that tropical enteropathy (contaminated bowel syndrome) is fairly frequent cause of chronic diarrhea, esp. in poor socio-economic strata, it will be justified to give a therapeutic trial on the lines of tropical sprue. We prefer to use

Table 3.10. Clinical features

	*Indian cases (150)**	*U.K. (52)***
Diarrhea	94	90
Failure to thrive	100	27
Anemia	100	14
Vomiting	20	61.5
Pain abdomen	20	45
Anorexia	46	50
Abdominal distension	73	44
Muscle wasting	53	14
Constipation	2	6

* Thapa et al. 1995 (All figures in percentage)

** Walker Smith et al., 1990.

cotrimoxazole (5 mg/kg/day of trimethoprim) and metronidazole (10-20 mg/kg/d) to try and suppress both aerobic and anaerobic bacteria, together with adequate nutritional advice. The response is seen within 15 days with control of diarrhea, restoration of appetite and improvement in weight. If this happens then treatment should be continued for about 12 weeks together with adequate dietary intake. After this the antibiotics can be stopped.

However, if this response is not seen within 15 days, then the antibiotics should not be continued and the child should be definitely referred for further work up to exclude celiac disease etc.

If celiac disease is diagnosed, management consists of complete withdrawal of gluten (wheat, rye, barley, oat). The diet should be completed with rice, maize, gram flour (*Besan*) etc. All care must be taken that flour of rice, maize and gram etc. are made in separate grinder so that even small amounts of wheat flour are not mixed, because even that can interfere with recovery. Legumes, milk products, vegetables and fruits can be taken liberally. However pickels (which contain "Rye") should be avoided. The response to gluten free diet in celiac disease, is seen within 4-6 weeks, but dietary therapy has to continue life long. Many of the fast foods and over the counter available foods may contain gluten, hence care must exercised in choosing these foods for these children. Dietary management of these children is quite complex and often frustrating. It is preferable that a pediatric gastroenterologist and a nutritionist are involved in the management.

In all cases of chronic diarrhea, it is most important to ensure adequate intake of a balanced diet. Supplementation with folic acid and zinc is helpful as also correction of anemia, if associated. The child's weight should be plotted on a growth chart and carefully followed up.

Bibliography

A manual for treatment of acute diarrhea, programme for control of diarrheal disease. World Health Organization, publication No. WHO/ODP/SER/80.2. Geneva.

Adachi, J.A. et al.: Enteroaggregative Esch. coli is a major etiologic agent in traveller's diarrhea in 3 regions of the world. Clin. Inf. Dis. 2001, 32 : 1706-1709.

Adani C.A. et al.: Antidiarrheal agents compared. Practice 1969, 202-269.

Alam, S. and Bhatnagar, S. Current status of anti-diarrheal and anti-secretory drugs in the management of childhood diarrhea. Ind. J. Ped., 2006, 73 : 693-696.

Alam, S. et al.: Dietary regimen for persistent diarrhea in infants under 4 months. Indian Pediatr. 2001, 38 : 396-400.

Amadi, B.: Role of food antigen elimination in treating children with persistent diarrhea and malnutrition in Zambia. J. Pediatr. Gastro. Nutr. 2002, 34 : (Suppl. 1) : S54-S56.

Avery G.B., Villavincencio, O., Litly, J.R. et al.: Intractable diarrhea in early infancy. Pediatrics 1968 : 41 : 712-722.

Awasthi, S., INCLEN Group. Zinc supplementation in acute diarrhea is acceptable, does not interfere with rehydration and reduces the use of other medication : a randomised trial in five countries. J. Ped. Gastro. Nutr., 2006, 42 : 300-305.

Baran, P., Tokne, G., Vagas, E., Oktean, S., Gokduma, M.K. Impact of zinc supplementation in children with acute diarrhea in Turkey. Arch. Dis. Child, 2006, 91 : 296-299.

Bhan, M.K., Khushoo, V., Sommerfelt, H. et al.: Entero-aggregative Escherichia coli and Salmonella associated with non-dysenteric persistent diarrhea. Ped. Inf. Dis. J. 1989, 8 : 499-502.

Bhan, M.K., Mahalanabis, D., Fontaine, O., Pierce, N. Clinical trials of improved ORS formulation : A Review. Bull WHO 1994, 72: 945-55.

Bhandari, N., Bahl, R., Taneja, S. et al. Substantial reduction in severe diarrheal morbidity by doing zinc supplementation in young north Indian children. Pediatr., 2002, 109 : e86.

Bhandari, N., Bhan, M.K. et al.: Mortality associated with acute watery diarrhea, dysentry and persistent diarrhea in north rural India. Acta. Pediatr. 1992, 81 (Sup. 381) : S36-S38.

Bhardwaj, A., Aggarwal, V., Chakraborty A., Mittal, S.K.: Does Rota virus infection cause persistent diarrhea. Trop. Gastroenterol. 1996, 17 : 18-21.

Bhatnagar, S., Bahl, R., Sharma, P.K. et al. Zinc with ORS reduces stool output and duration of diarrhea in hospitalised children : A randomised controlled trial. J. Pediat. Gastro. Nutr., 2004, 38: 34-40.

Bhatnagar, S., Bhan, M.K., Singh, K.D. et al.: Efficacy of milk-based diets in persistent diarrhea : A randomized controlled trial. Pediatr. 1996, 98 : 1127-36.

Bhatnagar, S., Bhandari, N., Mouli C., Bhan, M.K. IAP National Task Force. Consensus statement of IAP National Task Force:

Status Report on management of acute diarrhea. Ind. Pediat., 2004, 41 : 335-348.

Bhatnagar, S., Gupta, S.D., Mathur, M. et al. Celiac disease with mild to moderate histological changes is a common cause of chronic diarrhea in Indian children. J. Ped. Gastr. Nutr., 2005, 41 : 204-209.

Bhatnagar, S., Phillips, D and Bhan, M.K. Celiac disease in India. J. Pediatr. Gastro Nutr., 2006, 43 : 263-264.

Bhatnagar, S., Tandon, N. Diagnosis of Celiac Disease. Ind. J. Pediatr., 2006, 73 : 703-709.

Bhuta, Z.A., Hendricks, K.M.: Nutritional management of persistent diarrhea in childhood : A perspective from the developing world. J. Pediatr. Gastro. Nutr. 1996, 2 : 17-37.

Black, R.E., Sazawal, S.: Zinc and childhood infectious disease morbidity and mortality. Br. J. Nutr., 2001, 85 (Suppl 2) : S125-129.

Booth I.W., Levine, M.M., Harries, J.T. Oral rehydration therapy in acute diarrhea in childhood. J. Pediatr. Gastroenterol Nutr. 1984, 3 : 491-499.

Brooks, W.A., Santosham, M., Roy S.K. et al. Efficacy of zinc in young infants with acute watery diarrhea. Am. J. Clin. Nutri., 2005, 82 : 605-610.

Brown, K.H., Maclean, W.C. Jr. Nutritional Management of acute diarrhea : An appraisal of the alternatives, Pediatrics 1984, 73 : 119.

Caksen et al. Hyponatremic dehydration : An analysis of 78 cases. Int. Uro Nephro. 2001, 33 : 445-448.

Chen, L.C., Huq, E., Huffman, S.L. A Prospective study of the risk of diarrheal disease according to nutritional status of children. Am. J. Epidem. 1981, 114 : 284.

CHOICE study group. Multicentre, randomised, double-blind clinical trial to evaluate the efficacy and safety of a reduced osmolarity ORS in children with acute watery diarrhea. Pediatric, 2001, 107 : 613-618.

Chung, A.W., Viscorova, B. The effect of the early feeding versus early oral starvation on the course of infantile diarrhea. J. Pediatr. 1948; 33 : 14.

Cook, G.C. Post-infective malabsorption (including tropical sprue). In : Oxford Text Book of Medicine, 2nd edition. D.J. Weatherall, J.G.G. Leadingham and D.A. Warrel. Oxford Univ. Press, Oxford, 1987, pp. 12.115-12.120.

Dupont H.C. et al. Fecel leucocytes in Acute diarrhea. Indian Pediatr. 1984, 21.

Editorial Water with sugar and salt. Lancet 1978, 2 : 300-301.

Farthing, M.J.G. Oral Rehydration therapyl. Pharma therapy 1994, 64 : 477-492.

Fischer Walker, C.L., Bhuta, Z.A., Bhandari N. et al. Zinc supplementation for the treatment of diarrhea in infants in Pakistan, India and Ethiopia. J. Pediat. Gast. Nutr., 2006, 43 : 357-363.

Ghai, O.P. Jaiswal, V.N., Relationship of Undernutrition to diarrhea in infants and children. Indian J. Med. Res. 1970, 58 : 789-794.

Goldman, S.A., Anderson, D.W., Sellers, W.A. et al. Milk allergy I, oral challenges with milk and isolated milk protein in allergic children. Pediatr. 1963; 32 : 425-443.

Gupta, Vandita. Feasibility and efficacy of Gruels enriched with Amylase rich foods in the nutritional management of malnourished children with and without diarrhea. Thesis submitted to Delhi University for Ph.D. in Nutrition, 1996.

Haque, K.M., Binder, H.J. Zinc in treatment of acute diarrhea : Current Status and assessment. Gastroentero., 2006, 130 : 2201-05.

Hirschhorn, N., Kinzie, J.L., Sachar, D.B. et al. Decrease in net stool output in cholera during intestinal perfusion with glucose containing solutions. N. Engl. J., Med. 1968, 279 : 176-181.

Hoyle, B., Yunus, M., Chen, L.C. Breast feeding and food intake among children with acute diarrheal disease. Am. J. Clin. Nutr. 1980; 30 : 2365.

Iyangakaran, N., Robinson, N.T., Prathap, K. et al. Cow's milk protein sensitive enterolpathy : Combined clinical and histological criteria for diagnosis. Arch. Dis. child. 1978, 53 : 20-26.

Jackson, D., Walker Smith, J.A., Phillips, A.D. Macromolecular Absorptional by histologically normal and abnormal small Intestinal mucosa in childhood. An in vitro study using organ culture. J. Pediatr. Gastro. Nutr. 1983, 2 : 235-47.

Jhamb, U. Drug therapy in diarrhea in Update in pediatric Gastroenterology. Ed. S.K. Mittal, Ind. Acad. of Pediatrics, Delhi, 1986, pp. 61-71.

Karim, A.S. et al. Risk factors of persistent diarrhea in children below 5 yr. of age. Ind. J. Gastro, 2001, 20 : 59-61.

Kim, Y. Hahn, S. and Garner, P. Reduced osmolarity ORS for treating dehydration caused by acute diarrhea in children. Cochorane Database Syst. Rev. 2001(2) : CD002847. Update in Cochrane Database Rev. 2002 (1) CD002847.

Lebenthal, E. Prolonged small intestinal mucosal injury as a primary cause of intractable diarrhea of infancy. In : chronic diarrhea. Ed. E. Lebenthal. Nestle Nutrition Raven Press, New York, 1984, pp. 5-30.

Lima A.A. et al. Persistent diarrhea in Northeast Brazil : etiologies and interaction with malnutrition. Acta. Pedia., 1992, 81 : (Sup. 381) : S39-S44.

Mahalanabis, D., Merson, M. Development of an improved formulational of oral rehydrational salts (ORS) with anti-diarrheal and nutritional properties : A "Super ORS". In : Holmgren J. Lindberg A. Moll by R. Eds. Development of vaccines and Drugs against Diarrhea. 11th Nobel Conference, Stockholm, 1985. Student literature Sweden, 1986, pp. 240-256.

Mata, L. Epidemiology of acute diarrhea in childhood: An overview. In Acute Diarrhea : It's Nutritional consequences in children. Ed. Bellanti, J.A. Nestle, Vevey/Raven Press, New York, 1983, p. 1-18.

Mata, L., Kromal, R.A., Urrutia, J.J., Garcia, B. Effect of infection on food intake and the nutritional state : Perspective as viewed from village. Am. J. Clin. Nutr. 1977; 30 : 1215.

Mathan, V.I. Tropical sprue in Southern India. Trans R. Soc. Trop Med. Hyg. 1983, 82 : 10-14.

Meyers, P.W., Lermon, S. Rise and fall of Shigella antibiotic resistance. Antimicrob agents chemother. 1980 : 17 : 101-102.

Mittal, S.K. Universal oral rehydrational solution. Editorial Indian Pediatr., 1987.

Mittal, S.K., Saxena, S., Srivastav, G., Gupta, S. Acute diarrhea in malnourished children. Clinical, microbiological and biochemical profile. Indian Pediatr. 1980, 17.

Molla, A.M. and Molla, A. Nutritional management of diarrhea Update in Pediatric Gastroenterology, Ed. S.K. Mittal, Indian Academy of Pediatrics, Delhi, 1986, pp. 75-84.

Molla, A.M. et al. Rice based oral rehydration solution decrease stool volume in acute diarrheas. Bull WHO, 1985, 63 : 751-756.

Molla, A.M., Rahman, M., Sarkar, S.A., Sack, D.A., Moll, A. Stool electrolyte content and purging rates in diarrhea caused by rotavirus, enterotoxigenic E. Coli and V. cholera in children J. Pediatr., 1981, 96 : 835-838.

Morpeth, S.C., Thielman, N.M., Diarrhea in patients with AIDS.

Curr. Treatm. Options Gastroent. : 2006, 9 : 23-37.

Murphy, C., Hahn, S., Volmink, J. Reduced osmolarity ORS for treating children. Cochrane Database Syst. Rev., 2004, 18, CD003754 (Review).

Nagpal, J. and Gogia, S. Racecadotril. Ind. Pediatr., 2004, 41 : 1218-1224.

Nurku, S., Garcia-Ananrda, J.A., Fishein, F. et al. Successful use of chicken based diets for the treatment of severely malnourished children with persistant diarrhea : A prospective randomized study. J. Pediatr. 1997, 1312: 105-12.

Okeke, I.N., Natroo, J.P. Enteroaggregative E. coli. Lancet Infectious Diseases, 2001, 1 : 304-313.

Patel, P. et al. Fecel leucocytes in Acute diarrhea. Indian Pediatr., 1984, 21.

Pathak, A. Risk factors for persistent diarrhea. Thesis submitted to Delhi University for M.D. 1989.

Pathela, P., Zahid Hassan, K., Roy, E. et al. Diarrheal illness in a cohort of children 0-2 yrs of age in rural Bangladesh I. Incidence and risk factors. Acta. Pediat., 2006, 95 : 430-437.

Patwari, A.K., Anand, V.K., Aneja, S. and Sharma, D. Management of Persistent diarrhea in diarrheal Unit. Ind. Pediatr. 1995, 32 : 277-284.

Penny, M.E., Paredes, P.O., Brown, K.H. Clinical and Nutritional consequences of lactose feeding during persistent post enter Diarrhea. Pediatr. 1989; 84 : 835-844.

Poddar, U., Thapa, B.R., Singh, K. Clinical features of celiac disease in Indian children : Are they different from the West. J. Pediatr. Gastroenterol. Nutr., 2006, 43 : 313-317.

Portnoy, B.N. et al. Antidiarrheal agents in the treatment of acute diarrhea in children JAMA, 1976, 236 : 844.

Puri, A.S., Garg, S., Monga, R. et al. Spectrum of atypical celiac disease in India. Ind. Pediatr. 2004, 41 : 822-27.

Rahman, M.M. et al. Simultaneous zinc and vitamin A supplementation in Bangladeshi children. Randomised double blind trial. BMJ, 2001, 323 : 314-318.

Rahman, M.M., Mitra, A.K., Mahalanabis, D. et al. Absorption of nutrients from an energy dense diet liquified with amylase from germinated wheat in infant with acute diarrhea. J. Ped. Gastro. Nutr., 1997, 24 : 119-123.

Rajeshwari, K. and Mittal, S.K. Hypoosmotor, ORS. Pediatrics today, 1998, 1(2).

Ramsook, C., Shagun-Carrean, I., Kozinetz, C.A., Moro-Southerland, D. A randomised clinical trial comparing oral odensteron with placebo in children with vomiting from acute gastroenterits. Ann. Emerg. Med. 2002, 39 : 392-403.

Rhode, J. and Northrup, R.S. Diarrhea is a nutritional disease. Ind. Pediatr. 1988, 25 : 914-929.

Robson, A.M. Parenteral fluid therapy : in Text Book of Pediatrics Editors. W.E. Nelson, W.B. Saunders & Co. XIIth Edition, 1983, pp. 228-249.

Salazar-Lindo E., Santisteban-Ponce J., Chea-Woo E., Gutierrez, M. Racecadotril in the treatment of acute watery diarrhea in children. NEJM, 2000, 343 : 463-467.

Santha Krishnan, B.R., Uma Devi, L., Chronic protracted watery diarrhea in malnourished children. Ind. Pediatr. 1986 : 23 : 515-519.

Santosham, M., Fayad, I., Abu Zikri M. et al. A double blind clinical trial camparing WHO. ORS with a reduced osmolarity solution containing equal amounts of sodium and glucose. J. Pediat., 1996, 128 : 45-51.

Sarkar, S.A., Cass Wall, T.H., Mahalanabis, D. et al. Successful treatment of rota virus diarrhea in children with immunoglobulin from immunised bovine colostrum. Ped. Inf. Dis. J., 1998, 17 : 1149-54.

Sazawal, S., Bhan, M.K., Bhandor, N. Type of milk feeding during acute diarrhea and the risk of persistent diarrhea : A case control study. Acta. Pedia. (Suppl.) 1992, 381 : 93-97.

Silverman, A., Roy, C.C. Diarrheal disorders : In Pediatric Clinic Gastroenterology Eds. Silverman A, Roy C., St. Louis Toranto, London, C.V. Mosby Co., 1983, pp. 190-237.

Sood, A., Midha, V., Sood, N. et al. Prevalence of celiac disease among school children in Punjab, North India. J. Gastroenterol. Hepatol., 2006, 21 : 1622-1625.

Sullivan, P.B. Studies in small intestine in persistent diarrhea and malnutrition : the Gambia Exprience : J. Ped. Gastro. Nutr. 2002, 34 : (Suppl 1) : S11-13.

Tomkins, A. Nutritional status and severity of diarrhea among preschool children in rural Nigeria. Lancet, 1984, 1 : 860.

Tuinberg, L.A. Powell, D.W., Mahalanabis, D., Merson, M., Greenough W.B., Rabbonj, G.M. Prospects for improved rehydration therapy and antisecretory drug. In : Development of vaccines and drugs against diarrhea Eds. Jon Halmoren Londberg Alf, Mallby Ral Students Litteraurer, Lund, 1985, pp. 231-278.

Valentinor-Branth, P., Community based controlled trial of dietary management of children with persistent diarrhea: sustained beneficial effect on ponderal and linear growth. Am. J. Clin. Nutr. 2001, 73 : 968-974.

Walker Smith J.A. : Post-infectious diarrhea. Curr. Opin Inf. Dis. 2001, 14(5) : 567-571.

Walker Smith J.A., Nazer, H., Manual, P. et al. Protein intolerance as a cause of post enteritis diarrhea in Chronic Diarrhea Eds. Lebenthal. Raven Press N.Y. 1984, pp. 407-423.

WHO Bulletin. Persistent diarrhea in children in Developing Countries, 1988; 1-13.

WHO drug therapy in acute diarrhea 1996.

WHO, the management of Diarrhea and use of Oral Rehy dration Therapy. WHO/UNICEF statement, 2nd ed. World Health organisation, Geneva, 1985.

Yachha, S.K., Aggarwal, S., Srinivas, S. et al. Antibody testing in Indian children with celiac disease. Ind. J. Gastro., 2006, 25 : 132-135.